Endoscopic Sinus
Surgery Dissection Manual

Endoscopic Sinus Surgery Dissection Manual

A Stepwise, Anatomically Based Approach to Endoscopic Sinus Surgery

Roy R. Casiano

University of Miami School of Medicine
Miami, Florida

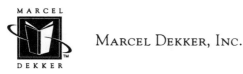

MARCEL DEKKER, INC.　　　　　　　　　　　NEW YORK · BASEL

ISBN: 0-8247-0743-5

Marcel Dekker, Inc., and the author make no warranty with regard to the accompanying software, its accuracy, or its suitability for any purpose other than as described in the preface. This software is licensed solely on an "as is" basis. The only warranty made with respect to the accompanying software is that the CD-ROM medium on which the software is recorded is free of defects. Marcel Dekker, Inc., will replace a CD-ROM found to be defective if such defect is not attributable to misuse by the purchaser or his agent. The defective CD-ROM must be returned within 10 days to: Customer Service, Marcel Dekker, Inc., P.O. Box 5005, Cimarron Road, Monticello, NY 12701, (914) 796-1919.

This book is printed on acid-free paper.

Headquarters
Marcel Dekker, Inc.
270 Madison Avenue, New York, NY 10016
tel: 212-696-9000; fax: 212-685-4540

Eastern Hemisphere Distribution
Marcel Dekker AG
Hutgasse 4, Postfach 812, CH-4001 Basel, Switzerland
tel: 41-61-261-8482; fax: 41-61-261-8896

World Wide Web
http://www.dekker.com

The publisher offers discounts on this book when ordered in bulk quantities. For more information, write to Special Sales/Professional Marketing at the headquarters address above.

Current printing (last digit):
10 9 8 7 6 5 4 3 2 1

PRINTED IN THE UNITED STATES OF AMERICA

To Sheila, Alex, Brendan, Briana, Christian,
and all the residents and fellows at the
Department of Otolaryngology–Head and Neck Surgery,
University of Miami School of Medicine.

Preface

This endoscopic sinus surgery (ESS) dissection manual illustrates a unique, anatomically based, and stepwise approach for learning to perform endoscopic sinus surgery. This approach has been used for years in teaching endoscopic surgical anatomy and technique to otolaryngology residents and fellows at the University of Miami School of Medicine. It combines all the best attributes of prior methodologies.

In this manual I illustrate how the bony ridge of the antrostomy and adjacent medial orbital floor can be very consistent and useful landmarks when performing ESS. By using the antrostomy ridge and medial orbital floor, in combination with columnellar measurements, even the most inexperienced surgeon can determine his or her approximate location within the ethmoid labyrinth and operate within a zone of confidence. Use of this approach also facilitates the determination of the correct anteroposterior trajectory into the posterior ethmoid and sphenoid sinuses. The methodical use of these landmarks keeps the surgeon oriented, especially when faced with significant anatomical distortion due to disease or prior surgery. That is, neither anatomical reference point appears to be significantly affected by inflammatory conditions or prior sinus surgery, and both are easy to find. Utilizing these consistent reference points minimizes the chance of inadvertent intracranial or intraorbital complications in the face of significant anatomical distortion.

The manual is divided into 20 dissections. Each of the dissections builds on the anatomical exposure and identification of key anatomical landmarks developed in the preceding dissection. In addition, an increasing degree of surgical skill and knowledge of the endoscopic paranasal sinus anatomy is required as the student progresses through all 20 dissections.

Therefore, one should complete each dissection before progressing to the next one in the manual. All the structures illustrated in each section should be completely identified. Remember that repetition is the key to developing an expertise in any surgical procedure. Finally, the endoscopic surgical skills acquired from this manual should be supplemented with additional reading from the references at the end of the manual to expand one's fund of knowledge in all the procedures discussed.

Roy R. Casiano

Contents

1

Consistent and Reliable Anatomical Landmarks in Endoscopic Sinus Surgery: A Historical Perspective

Transnasal sinus surgery began in 1886, when Miculicz reported on the endonasal fenestration of the maxillary sinus (1). A transnasal approach to performing an ethmoidectomy was not described until 1915, when Halle reported his experience (2). Even then, it was immediately apparent that a transnasal ethmoidectomy posed significant inherent risks for the patient. Indeed, these risks were best paraphrased by Mosher, in 1929, when he described intranasal ethmoidectomy as being "one of the easiest operations with which to kill a patient" (3). In the three decades that followed Mosher's work, a number of significant anatomical studies helped further define the three-dimensional anatomy and variations of the ethmoid labyrinth, turbinates, and surrounding ostia and recesses that drain the dependent sinuses (maxillary, frontal, and sphenoid) (4–10). Initially designed to evaluate the feasibility of irrigating the antrum via direct transnasal cannulation of the natural ostium, these studies contributed significantly to our current understanding of paranasal sinus endoscopic anatomy. They describe the wide variability in distances and dimensions among virtually all the intranasal anatomical structures currently used as landmarks in endoscopic sinus surgery (ESS).

The first attempt at nasal and sinus endoscopy was made by Hirshman in 1901, using a modified cystoscope (11). In 1925, Maltz, a New York rhinologist, used the term *sinoscopy* and advocated the technique for diagnosis (12). However, ESS was not introduced in the European literature until 1967, by Messerklinger (13). Moreover, it did not gain wider acceptance in Europe until others continued development and clarification of the technique (14–21). In 1985, Kennedy introduced the technique of functional endoscopic sinus surgery (FESS) into the United States (22). Since then, there has been an ongoing effort to refine the ESS technique and identify consistent anatomical landmarks to facilitate safe entry into the maxillary or sphenoid sinus, or to navigate within the ethmoid sinus (23–32).

Most rhinologists agree that ESS should be a "disease-directed" and mucosal-sparing operation, recognizing the principle of the potential for re-establishing drainage and mucosal recovery of the dependent sinuses (13,14,16). Since first described in 1965 by Neuman, the concept of the ostiomeatal unit, or complex, continues to play a role in mucosal disease of the paranasal sinuses (15). The ostiomeatal complex theory states that most inflammatory conditions of the maxillary, ethmoid, and frontal sinuses arise from this common drainage pathway. Therefore, the surgical procedure can be limited to an absolute minimum. Even in cases with significant radiological involvement of the frontal or maxillary sinuses, correction of ethmoid disease usually results in re-establishment of drainage and mucosal recovery of the larger (dependent) sinuses.

Today, there are essentially two techniques available to endoscopically address the ethmoid, maxillary, and sphenoid sinuses: the anteroposterior (AP) approach and posteroanterior (PA) approach (14,17,18,20). Anteroposterior exenteration of the ethmoid sinuses is the technique most widely used in the United States (14,17). The surgeon proceeds as far posteriorly as needed to remove diseased ethmoid cells and polyps and establish drainage only to the dependent sinuses that are blocked. In contrast, the posteroanterior approach is based on retrograde exposure of the ethmoid cells, beginning at the posterior ethmoids and sphenoid sinus and working in a posteroanterior direction along the skull base (18–20). The ethmoid cell septations are removed in a posteroanterior direction along the skull base and orbital wall using the roof and lateral wall of the sphenoid sinus as reference points for the superior and lateral limits of dissection, respectively.

In the AP approach, the surgeon begins with an anterior ethmoidectomy by removing the uncinate process, bullar cells, and agger nasi cells, and occasionally entering the frontal recess. The surgeon proceeds as far posteriorly as needed to remove diseased ethmoid cells and polyps. A limited maxillary antrostomy is typically not performed until after the ethmoid cells have been addressed. Bone is removed circumferentially (anteriorly toward the lacrimal duct and posteriorly toward the posterior fontanelle) to enlarge the maxillary ostium as needed. If a sphenoidotomy is indicated, a transethmoidal operation through the common wall of the sphenoid and posterior ethmoid sinus is described.

Proponents of the AP approach argue that even though it enables the surgeon to proceed as far posteriorly (into the posterior ethmoids or sphenoid) as needed, extensive surgery is infrequently indicated (14,17,22). However, not all surgeons share this view, arguing that patients with advanced nasal polyposis frequently have pansinus disease affecting not only the anterior ethmoids and dependent sinuses (maxillary and frontal) but also the sphenoethmoidal recess and surrounding ostia draining the posterior ethmoids and sphenoid sinuses (33). Also, the AP approach assumes that the inexperienced surgeon will correctly identify critical anatomical structures such as the uncinate process, ostium of the maxillary sinus, middle and superior turbinate and surrounding recesses, the basal lamella of the middle and superior turbinates, the anterior ethmoid artery and anterior skull base, and the anterior and posterior ethmoid air cells. The surgeon is taught to identify these structures and to stay "inferomedially" as he or she progresses posteriorly to minimize the chances of inadvertently penetrating the orbital wall or skull base. The problem for the inexperienced surgeon is that often these structures are missing or distorted because of pathological conditions or prior surgery. In addition, during the course of the surgical procedure, the nasal telescope and/or camera may become rotated within the nose. The unsuspecting surgeon may think he or she is heading in an inferoposterior direction while in fact following a superior or lateral trajectory toward the skull base or orbit. In the absence of other consistent anatomical landmarks as internal reference points, the surgeon may fail to see that he or she is improperly oriented and that the skull base descends posteroinferiorly (34). This may result in inadvertent penetration of the anterior skull base or orbit as the AP ethmoidectomy is performed.

To address the difficulties observed when performing a sphenoidotomy using the traditional AP approach, Parsons described his approach to the sphenoid sinus (29). An anterior and posterior ethmoidectomy is performed (as with the AP approach) and the superior turbinate is visualized. The natural ostium of the sphenoid sinus is visualized on the medial side of the superior turbinate. A measurement is obtained from the natural ostium of the sphenoid to the anterior nasal spine. The same measuring instrument is then placed through the operative field, lateral to the middle and superior turbinates, to the "suspected" posterior wall of the posterior ethmoid. The second measurement has to be equal to or greater than the first measurement (at the natural ostium) for the suspected wall to qualify as the real anterior wall of the sphenoid sinus and not a posterior wall or a suprasphenoidal (Onodi) cell. A rigid instrument, such as a straight suction tip, is placed in the inferomedial quadrant. The instrument is advanced as far posterior and inferomedially as the dissection will allow. The surgeon then sweeps the suction tip medially toward the septum. According to Parsons, the bony wall of the superior/supreme turbinate will fracture in a very "consistent fashion," exposing a near vertical fracture line, which he refers to as the "ridge." The surgeon continues to sweep the superior turbinate medially, exposing the lateral mucosa of the superior turbinate medial to the ridge, referred to as the "ethmoid fontanelle," thereby visualizing the natural ostium of the sphenoid sinus.

Like other modifications of the AP approach, Parsons' technique has significant flaws due to some erroneous assumptions. He assumes that most surgeons performing a total ethmoidectomy can correctly identify, in the presence of inflammatory conditions, the sphenoid natural ostium, the middle and superior turbinates, and the posterior wall of the posterior ethmoid. He further assumes that the surgeon will be able to safely perform an anterior and posterior ethmoidectomy, identify the "ridge" as described, and introduce the suction tip correctly "inferomedially" into the sphenoid sinus. Blindly "advancing" suction tips (or today, power instrumentation) into any cavity can yield disastrous consequences. The inexperienced surgeon may face orientation difficulties with respect to how far inferomedially he or she has to be.

In 1999, Bolger and colleagues also tried to address the difficulties in consistently and safely opening the sphenoid sinus using the AP approach (30). Like Parsons, Bolger noted that identification of the superior meatus and superior turbinates provides a reliable landmark within the dissection field that can facilitate the surgical identification of the sphenoid sinus. He advises resecting 2–3 mm of the inferior and medial aspect of the basal lamella of the middle turbinate, and notes that little has been written about an endoscopic approach to the sphenoid sinus that uses this "discrete, easily identifiable, and reliable anatomic landmark." Bolger describes a "parallelogram-shaped box": medially the lateral aspect of the superior turbinate and, when present, the supreme turbinate; laterally the lamina papyracea; superiorly the skull base; and inferiorly the horizontal portion of the superior turbinate as it courses to attach to the lateral nasal wall. The back of this box is the anterior wall of the sphenoid sinus. Bisecting the box with a line connecting the superomedial corner to the inferolateral corner forms two triangles. Dissection in the inferomedial triangular region will be safe, whereas dissection in the superolateral triangular region will be hazardous because of the proximity of the optic nerve and the carotid artery. Just as Parsons and his coworkers had, the authors of this study found the superior meatus and the inferior aspect of the superior turbinate (unlike the middle turbinate) to be a consistent and reliable anatomical landmark for the location of the sphenoid sinus that is rarely resected with prior surgery. However, like Parsons' technique, this approach relies on the surgeon's ability to perform a complete ethmoidectomy with correct identification of the lamina papyrecea and anterior skull base anterior to this point. In addition, most inexperienced surgeons often find that distortion due to scarring or inflammatory disease often makes it very difficult to reliably identify the remnant of the superior turbinate.

Despite Parsons' and Bolger's attempts to address the difficulties with safely and consistently identifying the sphenoid sinus through a transethmoidal (AP) approach, significant problems remain. First, a transethmoidal sphenoidotomy does not always afford optimal access: the bone of the anterior wall of the sphenoid is thicker than that paramedially adjacent to nasal septum in the area of the sphenoid natural ostium (31). Since this procedure is carried out relatively close to the optic nerve and the carotid artery, specific anatomical variations in these skull-base structures may preclude the use of these techniques because of the potential for significant complications. Second, anatomical characteristics, such as a deviated nasal septum, may force the surgeon to take a more lateral trajectory into the sphenoid sinus, which, without a consistent reference point for initial entry into the sphenoid, requires a great deal of experience. The unwary surgeon can easily misjudge the appropriate level of entry into the sphenoid or posterior ethmoid and inadvertently enter the skull base, carotid artery, or optic nerve. Lastly, if the osteomeatal complex theory also applies to the sphenoethmoidal recess and surrounding ostia to the posterior sinuses ("posterior osteomeatal complex" to the sphenoid and posterior ethmoids), then whichever endoscopic surgical technique is selected must also address the natural drainage areas of these sinuses. In other words, the natural ostium of the sphenoid needs to be enlarged rather than a new one created through the common wall of the sphenoid and posterior ethmoid sinus. The transethmoidal technique does little to ensure that the natural ostium is incorporated into the surgical sinusotomy (as is commonly done with the maxillary sinus ostium).

For these reasons, a sphenoidotomy adjacent to the nasal septum and *medial* to the superior turbinate has been proposed (26,31,32). Any bleeding during enlargement of the sphenoid ostium inferiorly can be easily controlled with cautery. Hosemann et al. note that perforation of the anterior sphenoid wall 10–12 mm superior to the choanal arch in the area of the natural ostium, as described by Wigand, is the preferable strategy (31). This point corresponds to the middle third of the anterior sphenoid sinus wall in 88% of the cases and to the superior third in the remainder.

Recognizing the potential difficulties with the AP approach, especially with more extensive disease of the paranasal sinuses, Wigand described the PA approach (18–20). In this approach, the surgeon opens the sphenoid beginning with a posterior partial resection of the middle turbinate. The posterior ethmoid sinus is opened by limited removal of the posterior free body of the middle turbinate. The sphenoid is entered by using a suction tip with gentle pressure 1–2 cm above the upper edge of the posterior nasal choanal arch. Wigand notes that his technique poses little danger of perforating the skull base because the rigid plate of the sphenoid planum will be encountered if the surgeon goes too high. Nevertheless, he advises against exposing the posterior ethmoid cells as far as the ethmoid roof at this point. Rather, he advocates first exposing and removing the anterior wall of the sphenoid sinus to avoid dissection toward the skull base. Once the roof of the sphenoid and lateral wall are identified (as the superior and lateral limits of dissection, respectively), a retrograde dissection of the ethmoid cells is performed. Wigand describes performing an antrostomy last through the posterior fontanelle since this is a consistent reference point for safely entering the maxillary sinus.

According to Wigand, the PA approach gives a clear exposure of the surgical field, reducing the risk of serious complications and yielding reliable results without long-term crusting. This approach, however, is more extensive than the AP approach, irrespective of the extent of the disease.

It is usually combined with a septoplasty (to ensure medial entry into the sphenoid) and involves routine opening of the sphenoid, frontal, and maxillary sinuses (a pansinus operation). It also requires a certain degree of precision and experience in determining the exact location of the sphenoid sinus in the sphenoethmoidal recess. With advanced disease, the anatomy in this area may be significantly distorted. As with the AP approach, the superior or middle turbinate may be difficult to identify. There is also great variability when relying on internal measurements alone. The mean distance from the choanal arch to the sphenoid ostium is 8 mm (range 2–15 mm) (31). The mean distance from the sphenoid ostium to the skull base is also 8 mm (range 3–17). In addition, the sphenoid ostium can be even closer to the posterior cribriform plate than the skull base (approximately 3 mm) (6). As previously noted, anatomical characteristics such as a deviated nasal septum may force the surgeon to take a more lateral trajectory into the sphenoid sinus, which requires a great deal of experience. Moreover, in the event of inadvertent penetration, the use of suction tips (as advocated by Wigand) could further enhance the trauma by contusing brain parenchyma and other neural structures.

In 1994, May and colleagues introduced six friendly anatomical landmarks that are almost always present despite previous surgery: 1) the arch (or convexity) formed by the posterior edge of the lacrimal bone, 2) the anterior superior attachment of the middle turbinate, 3) the middle meatal antrostomy and the bony "ridge" along its superior border formed by the junction of the floor of the orbit with the lamina papyracea and posterior fontanelle, 4) the lamina papyracea, 5) the nasal septum, 6) and the arch of the posterior choana (27). Using these landmarks, revision ESS for recurrent or persistent disease in the maxillary, ethmoid, sphenoid, or frontal sinuses can be safely performed. May was one of the first to acknowledge that in advanced sinus disease anatomical landmarks such as the uncinate process, basal lamina, and superior or middle turbinate are not always readily identifiable. He was also one of the first to point out that the floor of the orbit, as seen through an antrostomy, serves as a consistent landmark from which other structures may be found. The bony "ridge" of the antrostomy represents the approximate level of the floor of the orbit as it inclines superiorly toward the orbital apex. This ridge is a useful landmark in identification of the lamina papyracea and in locating the posterior ethmoid and sphenoid sinuses. The posterior ethmoid sinus is located above this ridge and the sphenoid sinus lies below it. When a maxillary antrostomy is not performed, the natural ostium of the maxillary sinus can be alternatively used to help define the level of the orbit floor. The internal maxillary ostium is found at the junction of the medial maxillary wall and the floor of the orbit, halfway between the anterior and posterior maxillary walls and behind the convexity of the nasolacrimal duct.

Despite prior reports that showed great intersubject variability, May and Stankiewicz reintroduced the possible clinical efficacy of using standard measurements from the columnella to orient the surgeon during ESS (28,32). They based this proposal on anecdotal experience and prior anatomical studies by others noting that the distance from the area of the anterior nasal spine to the sphenoid ostium is approximately 60 mm (range 47–70 mm) (6,35,36). Adding approximately one more centimeter for the length of the columnellar base would make the mean distance to the sphenoid ostium around 70 mm. For this reason, May advocates labeling instruments with colored tape to warn the surgeon when the anterior face of the sphenoid is reached (approximately 7 cm). However, there will likely be variability among surgeons' measurements of these distances. In isolation, these measurements have not been shown to be clinically reliable. Until recently there have been no studies looking at the columnellar to sphenoid (or posterior ethmoid) measurement as a reference point when used by itself or in combination with other, more consistent anatomical landmarks.

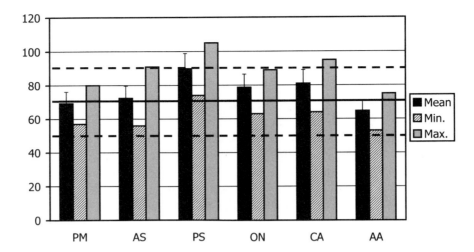

Figure 1 Graph illustrating the minimum, maximum, and mean distances (in mm) and standard deviations (bars) from the columnellar base to the posterior wall of the maxillary sinus (PM), anterior wall of the sphenoid sinus (AS), posterior wall of the sphenoid sinus (PS), distal canalicular portion of the optic nerve (ON), carotid artery (CA), and anterior ethmoid artery (AA). The dotted lines (50 and 90 mm) represent the zone of safety. The solid black line (70 mm) represents the critical measurement for accessing the sphenoid sinus.

More recently, Schaefer was the first to described a "hybrid technique" that combines the conservation goals of the AP approach with the anatomical virtues of the PA approach (26). Surgery begins with identification and complete removal of the uncinate process. If further surgery of the ethmoid sinus is warranted, the maxillary natural ostium is enlarged posteriorly or inferiorly rather than anteriorly to avoid injury to the lacrimal canal. Schaefer notes that this immediately exposes the level of the orbital floor. Like May, Schaefer recognizes the importance of the medial orbital floor as a landmark to facilitate identification of the inferior lamina papyrecea prior to proceeding with an ethmoidectomy. Schaefer advocates removal of the inferior two-thirds of the ethmoid cells in an AP direction using a 0-degree telescope. Often this involves removal of most, if not all, of the basal lamella of the middle turbinate to address the drainage area of the posterior sinuses and to facilitate entry into the sphenoid sinus. If indicated, the sphenoid sinus is entered inferior to the superior turbinate, at a plane between the middle turbinate and nasal septum. If the ostium cannot be visualized or palpated, the sphenoid is entered in the inferomedial quadrant of the anterior wall of the sinus. This approach ensures that the surgeon will maintain a safe distance from the skull base. After the surgeon identifies the sphenoid sinus roof, the superior extent of dissection is determined and the ethmoidectomy is completed more superiorly using a 30-degree telescope.

Schaefer's approach, like May's, recognizes the importance of performing an antrostomy prior to an ethmoidectomy to identify the orbital floor and medial orbital wall. Schaefer was the first to note the importance of performing an inferior ethmoidectomy before proceeding posteriorly, recognizing that this directs the surgeon safely away from the skull base as the orbital wall is followed posteriorly. As the surgeon proceeds posteriorly, it is the orbital wall that dictates the trajectory and not some ill-defined and often distorted lamella or turbinate structure, as advocated

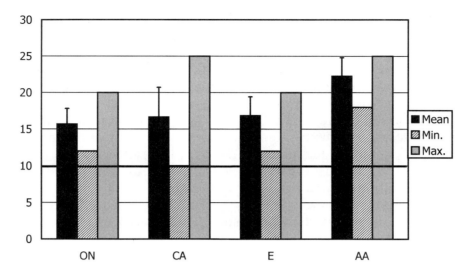

Figure 2   Graph illustrating minimum, maximum, and mean distances (in mm) and standard deviations (bars) from the antrostomy ridge and adjacent MOF to the optic nerve (ON), carotid artery (CA), roof of the ethmoid (E), and anterior ethmoid artery (AA). The solid black line (10 mm) represents the initial safe distance from the medial orbital floor, as seen through a middle meatal autrostomy, when performing an ethmoidectomy.

by proponents of the AP approach. It is only after the sphenoid roof has been identified that a superior dissection of the ethmoid cavity (if indicated) is performed, as with the PA approach.

Schaefer's study does not, however, define the vertical extent of the initial "inferior ethmoidectomy" from the level of the medial floor of the orbit. Mosher has shown that the height of the ethmoid labyrinth ranges from 2.5 to 3 cm (3); however, this height may vary even more depending on whether it is measured anteriorly or posteriorly. Similarly, the distance of two-thirds of the ethmoid cells, as described by Schaefer, can be quite variable. The maximum vertical distance permitted for an "inferior ethmoidectomy" as the surgeon proceeds posteriorly before critical skull-base structures are at risk remains unclear. Similarly, the level of the initial penetration (superiorly or inferiorly) into the sphenoid if the superior or middle turbinates are absent or distorted is open to interpretation. As with the AP approach, entering blindly through the "inferior and medial quadrant" of the anterior sphenoid wall does not clearly define the appropriate point of entry.

Despite their practical clinical utility, May's and Schaefer's observations are limited by the lack of studies to confirm the consistency or reliability of their measures through endoscopic means. Also, it is not clear how consistent the distance from the medial orbital floor is from the critical orbital or skull-base structures and how this landmark can be better used to facilitate endoscopic surgical orientation.

In 2001, Casiano confirmed May's and Schaefer's observations on a series of human cadavers (37). In this study, two examiners, with varying experience in endoscopic sinus surgery, performed endoscopic and direct measurements from the columnella and medial orbital floor to critical orbital and skull-base structures. The distances to four critical skull-base or orbital structures (the carotid artery, optic nerve, mid-ethmoid roof, and anterior ethmoid artery), and to the anterior and posterior wall of the sphenoid sinus, were measured. The mean, ranges, and standard deviations for all measurements (endoscopic and direct) were calculated. In addition, the variability in measurements between examiners and between the endoscopic and direct measurements was also determined.

The author found that the mean and range of values for each of the variables correlated well both between examiners and between endoscopic and direct measurements. The columnellar measurements (Figure 1) appeared to be very consistent between examiners and between endoscopic and direct measurements. When the antrostomy ridge and adjacent medial orbital floor was used (Figure 2), there was some slight variability between the individual measurements of the examiners and between endoscopic and direct measurements. However, the differences in measurements were no more than a few millimeters and did not appear to affect the overall clinical utility of these values. Casiano concluded that the bony ridge of the antrostomy and adjacent medial orbital floor, when combined with the use of columnellar measurements, are easily identifiable and consistent anatomical landmarks that provide even the most inexperienced surgeon with reliable information to navigate through even the most distorted paranasal sinus cavities.

2

Surgical Instrumentation, Setup, and Patient Positioning

A. Surgical Instrumentation (Figures 3 and 4)

Very few instruments are actually required to perform ESS. However, as one gains more surgical experience, there may be a need for additional instrumentation depending on the type of procedure or on the surgeon's personal preferences. The minimum instrumentation required for most of the dissections in this manual include: 1) a 30-degree telescope, 2) a 360-degree backbiting forceps, 3) a 360-degree sphenoid punch or forceps, 4) a 4-mm-long curved suction, 5) a 10 or 12 French straight (Frazier) suction with calibrated centimeter markings, 6) a 3.5-mm straight through-cut forceps, 7) a 3.5-mm upbiting through-cut forceps, 8) a small angled ball probe, and 9) a Cottle periosteal elevator. Powered instrumentation with a 4-mm straight and/or 60-degree cannula can be used in lieu of forceps to perform an ethmoidectomy and multiple sinusotomies.

For more advanced procedures, a 70-degree telescope is useful to visualize lateral or superior recesses of the frontal, maxillary, or sphenoid sinus. Curettes of various sizes are useful for removing thick bone, especially around the frontal ostium or sphenoid rostrum. Powered instrumentation with cutting or diamond burrs may also be necessary to carefully remove bone around critical structures such as the lacrimal sac, skull base, optic nerve, or carotid artery.

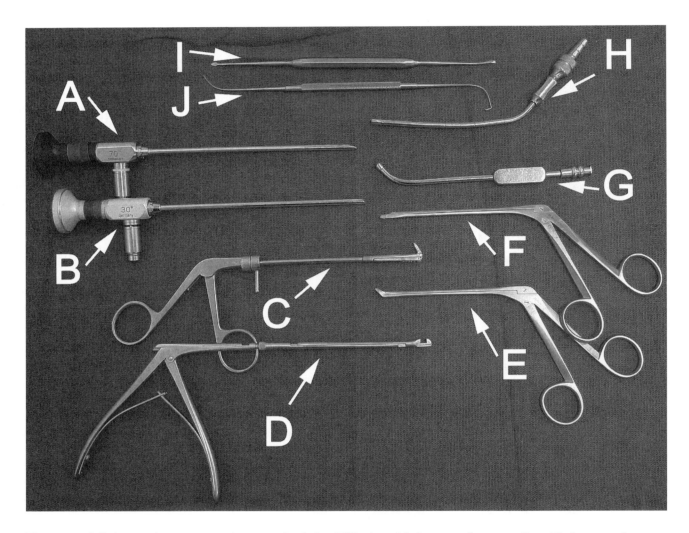

Figure 3 Minimum instrumentation required for ESS. A = 30-degree telescope. B = 70-degree telescope (optional). C = 360-degree backbiting forceps. D = 360-degree sphenoid punch or forceps. E = 3.5-mm upbiting through-cut forceps. F = 3.5-mm straight through-cut forceps. G = 4 mm long curved suction. H = calibrated straight (Frazier) suction. I = Cottle periosteal elevator. J = ostium seeker or ball probe, which is angled at one end and curved at the other.

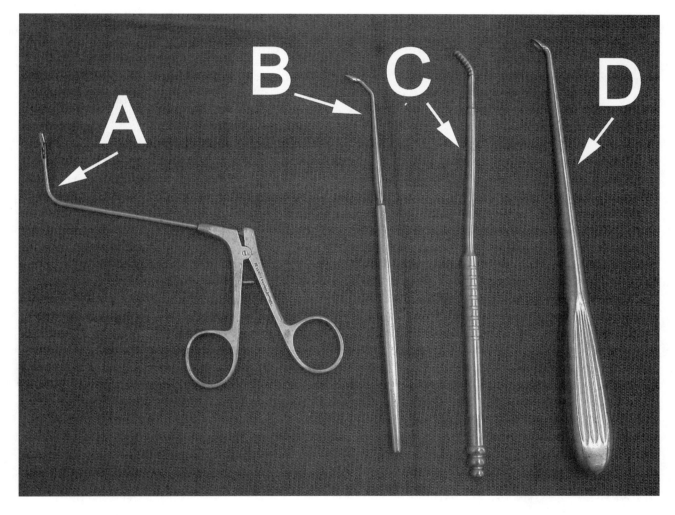

Figure 4 Additional instrumentation required for bone and tissue removal around the frontal ostium or sphenoid rostrum area. These instruments can be useful when performing an extended frontal or sphenoid sinusotomy. A = giraffe forceps. B = frontal curette. C = frontal rasp. D = angled cervical spine curette.

B. OR Setup and Patient Positioning (Figures 5–10)

The surgeon should be sitting or standing comfortably at the patient's side. A right-handed surgeon typically stands on the right side of the patient and a left-handed surgeon stands on the left side of the patient. If the surgeon chooses to sit, then a Mayo stand (cushioned with a pillow) is used to rest the arm holding the telescope at a comfortable height over the patient's head. The video tower and any intraoperative imaging devices are positioned at the head of the table, facing the surgeon.

A clear adhesive dressing (e.g., OpSite) is placed over the eye for protection. This allows the surgeon to visualize and palpate the eyes during the surgical procedure. The patient's face is draped to expose only the forehead, eyes, nose, and upper lip. The mouth and endotracheal tube are typically draped out unless a concomitant sublabial or oral procedure is planned.

The manner in which the telescope is grasped or instrumentation introduced into the nose may vary depending on the surgeon's personal preference, the specific length and type of telescope

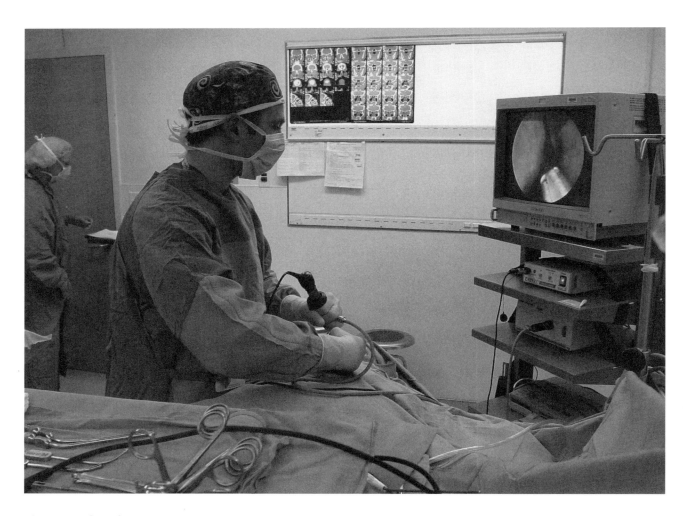

Figure 5   Standing position.

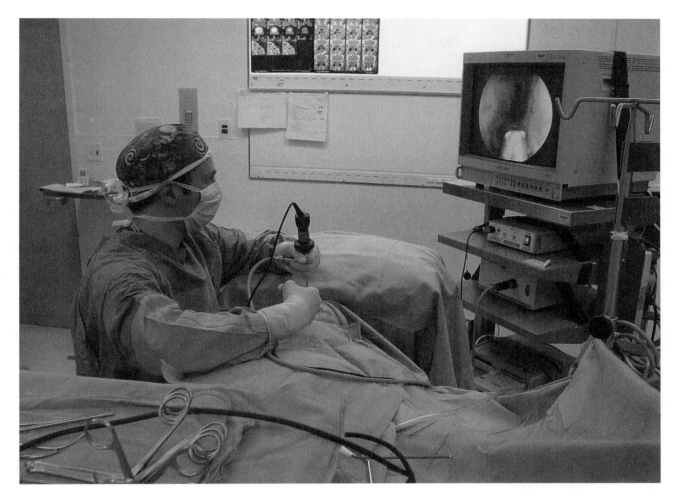

Figure 6   Sitting position, resting the elbow on a Mayo stand.

and/or camera, and the specific anatomical area being addressed. Generally, the surgeon determines which manner is best suited for his or her own hand.

A 30-degree telescope looking laterally is all that is typically necessary for most of the dissections described in this manual. A 0-degree telescope may also be used, but may limit adequate visualization of the lateral nasal structures (i.e., maxillary natural ostium, maxillary sinus, supraorbital ethmoidal cells, etc.). The axis of the telescope is directed toward the occipital area of the head and the superior border of the inferior turbinate is kept in view during the initial part of the procedure until the medial orbital floor is identified through the antrostomy. This keeps the surgeon directed toward the choanal arch and superior nasopharynx. The telescope is positioned at the nasoseptal angle with gentle superior retraction of the nasal tip and the surgical instrumentation is inserted inferior to the telescope.

A 70-degree telescope can be used if further visualization is required into the superior or lateral recesses of the frontal, maxillary, or sphenoid sinus. The 30-degree or 70-degree telescope is placed along the floor of the vestibule looking superiorly (as when working around the frontal ostium) or medially (as when performing a septoplasty). In these cases, the instruments are introduced superior to the telescope.

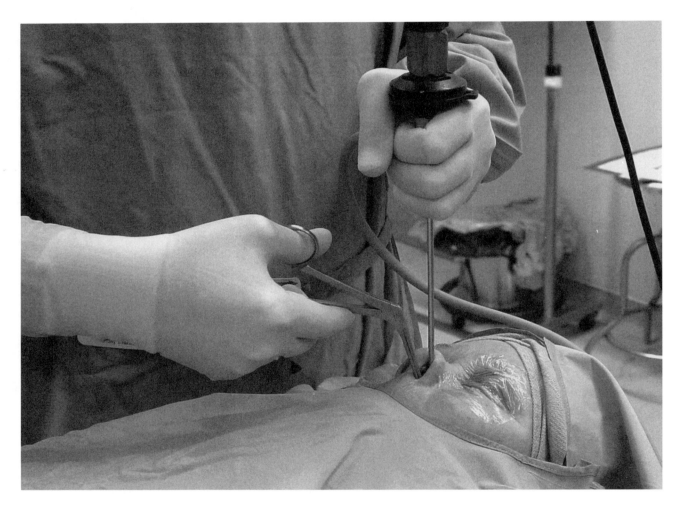

Figure 7 The telescope is grasped comfortably and the instrumentation is introduced inferior to the telescope for most of the procedures.

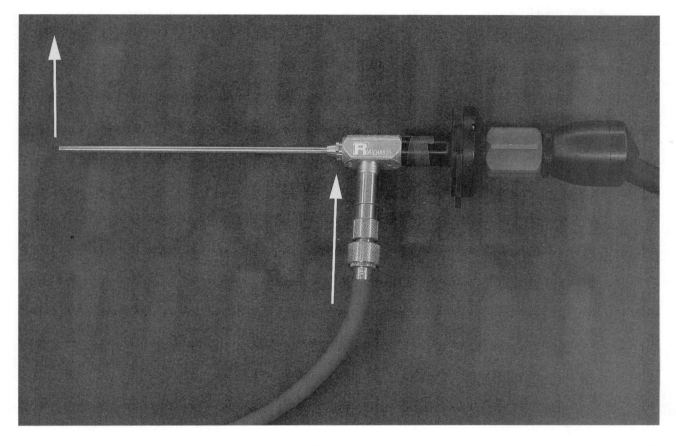

Figure 8   The direction that the surgeon is visualizing through an angled telescope corresponds to the direction in which the fiberoptic light cable enters the telescope (arrows). This is one way the surgeon can tell which direction he or she is looking at while performing ESS.

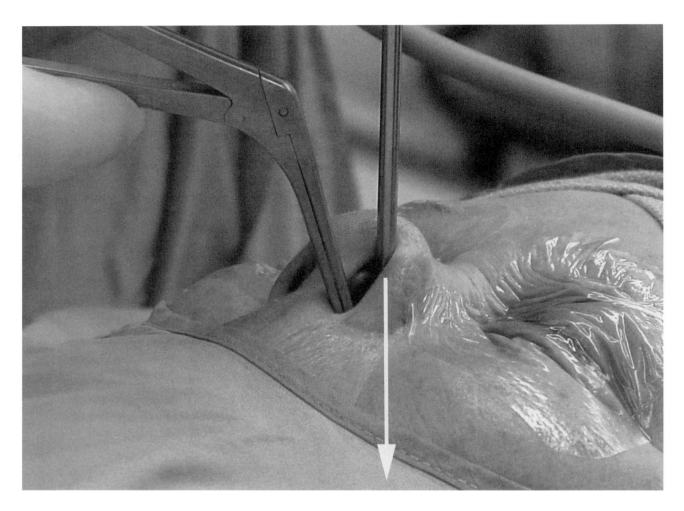

Figure 9 For most of the dissections the 30-degree telescope is directed toward the patient's occipital area (arrow), with gentle superior retraction of the nasal tip and ala.

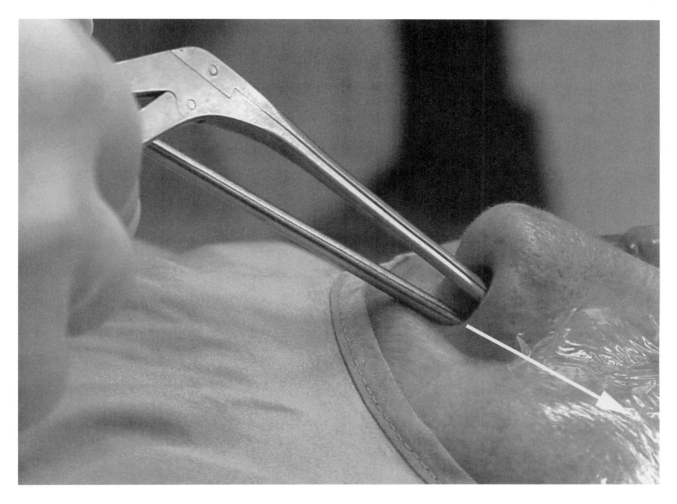

Figure 10   The instrumentation is introduced superior to the telescope when working around the frontal ostium.

3

Basic Dissection

A. Intranasal Examination (Figure 11)

The structures of the posterior nasal choana (i.e., the eustachian tube opening, choanal arch, posterior septum, and posterior nasopharyngeal wall), along with the inferior turbinate, are routinely identified with a 0-degree or 30-degree telescope before proceeding with endoscopic surgery of the paranasal sinuses. Identification of these structures early on establishes the anteroposterior dimensions of the nasal airway, provides a drainage route for blood into the nasopharynx, and facilitates the introduction of endoscopic surgical instrumentation and telescopes. Hypertrophied middle and/or inferior turbinates, and/or a septal spur or deviation obstructing the nasal airway or limiting endoscopic exposure, are addressed prior to proceeding with any sinus work. When bilateral polyp disease is present, a bilateral nasal polypectomy is performed first to re-establish the anteroposterior dimensions of the nose, as well as to facilitate the placement of a contralateral nasopharyngeal suction.

Hemostasis and adequate nasal exposure and evacuation of blood are imperative, especially when addressing advanced inflammatory disease of the nose and paranasal sinuses. A separate contralateral suction is used for the continuous evacuation of accumulated blood and debris from the nasopharynx. The nose is topically decongested and infiltrated with vasoconstrictive agents. Monopolar or bipolar suction cautery is helpful if discrete bleeding vessels are encountered during surgery. However, excessive cauterization should be avoided to minimize crusting and prolonged healing in these areas.

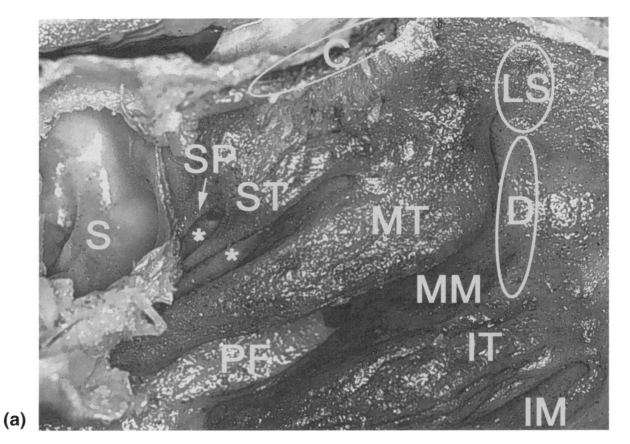

(a)

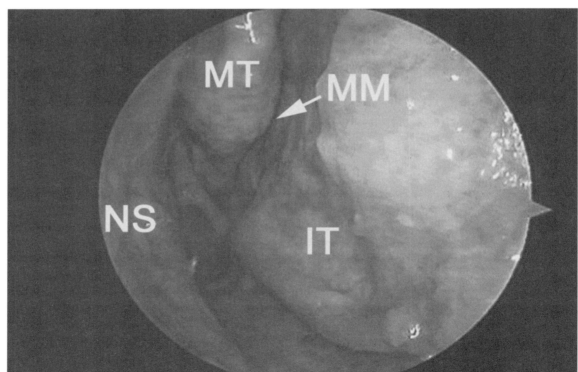

(b)

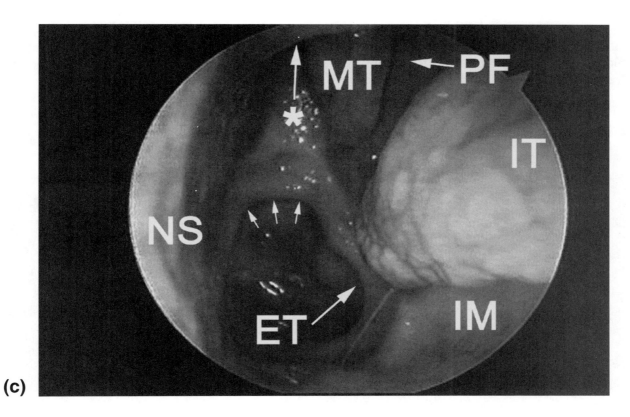

Figure 11 Sagittal (a) and endoscopic (b and c) views of the internal nasal structures. IT = inferior turbinate. MT = middle turbinate. ST = superior turbinate. SP = supreme turbinate. IM = inferior meatus. MM = middle meatus. Asterisks = sphenoethmoidal recess. LS = lacrimal sac. D = lacrimal duct. PF = posterior fontanelle. NS = nasal septum. ET = eustachian tube orifice. Small arrows in the endoscopic view denote the posterior choanal arch.

B.   Inferior Turbinoplasty (Figure 12)

An endoscopic inferior turbinoplasty may be indicated when there is poor endoscopic visualization of the nasal and posterior choanal structures or nasal obstruction due to turbinate hypertrophy (38,39). Frequently, the turbinate bone is the primary cause of turbinate hypertrophy and nasal obstruction (40). The inferior edge of the inferior turbinate, adjacent to the nasal floor, is incised or de-epithelialized to expose the turbinate bone along its entire extent with a 30-degree telescope looking slightly superolaterally. A medial mucosal flap is raised and the turbinate bone is partially or totally removed in a piecemeal fashion. To minimize the chance of secondary maxillary sinusitis, care should be taken to avoid fracturing the inferior turbinate lamellar attachment to the lateral nasal wall (41). For additional airway space, the lateral (inferior meatal) mucosal flap is trimmed as needed. At the completion of the procedure, the medial and lateral mucosal flaps are reapposed along the entire anteroposterior extent of the inferior turbinate. This minimizes the chance of prolonged crusting due to exposed bone (osteitis) or de-epithelialized surfaces.

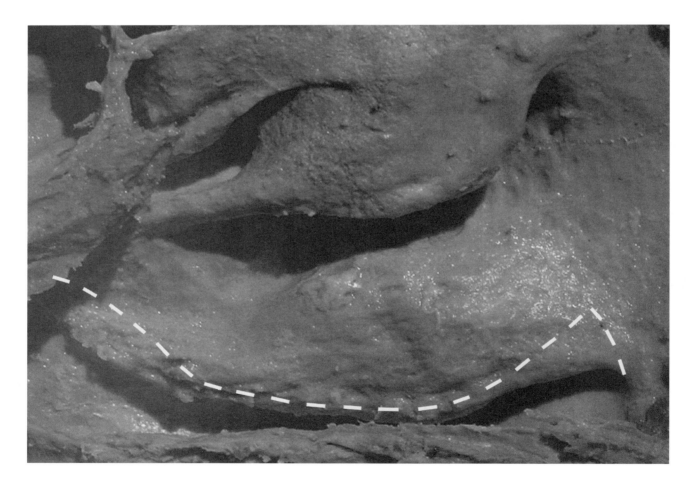

Figure 12   Dotted line demarcates the incision for an inferior turbinoplasty. This can be performed with a cutting forceps, sickle knife, or powered instrumentation.

C. Septoplasty (Figures 13 and 14)

A significant septal spur or deviation may preclude adequate endoscopic visualization or adversely affect nasal airway patency. In these cases an endoscopic septoplasty may be indicated (42–45). An endoscopic septoplasty begins with the elevation of an L-shaped posterosuperiorly based mucoperiochondrial flap. The 30-degree telescope is rotated to look slightly superomedially. Care is taken to place the vertical portion of the incision immediately anterior to the deviated area to facilitate cartilage or bone removal. The mucosal incision should be made only through the mucosa on the ipsilateral side. The horizontal portion of the incision is made perpendicular to the vertical incision at the junction of the floor and nasal septum or just slightly superior to this point, depending on the extent of the deviation. The contralateral mucoperichodrium is identified and preserved, especially at the incision area, to avoid the chance of a permanent septal perforation. The septal spur or deviated portion of the nasal septum is removed and the mucoperichondrial

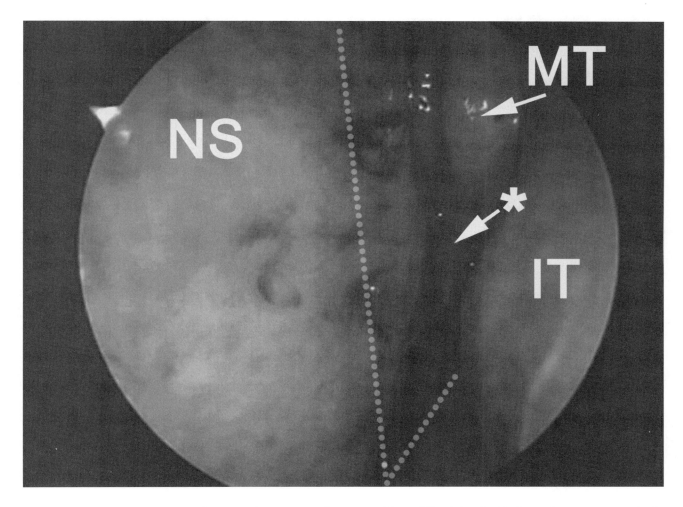

Figure 13 Endoscopic view showing the proposed incision (dotted line) for the L-shaped posterosuperiorly based mucoperichondrial flap. NS = nasal septum. MT = middle turbinate. IT = inferior turbinate. Asterisk denotes a septal spur.

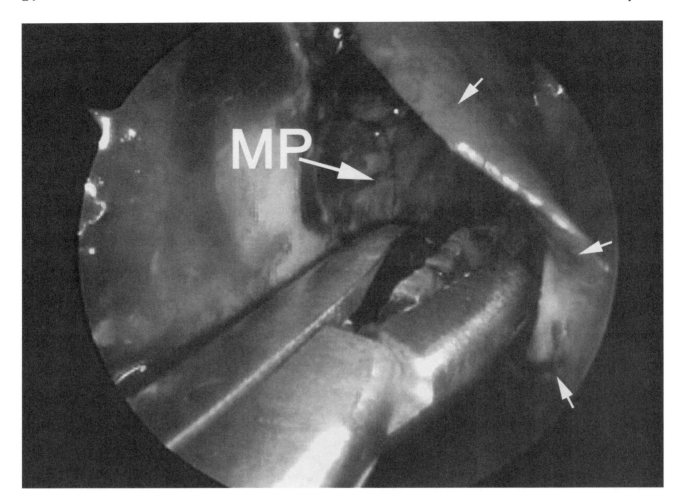

Figure 14 Endoscopic view showing the ipsilateral mucoperichondrial flap (arrows) is elevated toward the inferior turbinate. Bone or cartilage is carefully removed while preserving the contralateral mucoperichondrium (MP).

flap is returned to its normal position. Occasionally it is necessary to remove a strip of perpendicular plate cartilage or bone inferior to the rhinion area in order to free up a caudal deflection. Nevertheless, a dorsal and caudal strut of septal cartilage is always preserved to avoid the chance of septal collapse and saddle-nose deformity. At the conclusion of the procedure, the vertical septal incision may be sutured, although this is usually not necessary unless the flap interferes with the introduction of the telescope or instruments. Otherwise, blood is allowed to drain through the horizontal incision to minimize the chance of hematoma formation. Packing or basting sutures are generally not required unless the septal incisions are sutured.

D. Middle Turbinoplasty (Figures 15 and 16)

When the middle turbinate is enlarged, a middle turbinoplasty may be indicated (46,47). Middle turbinate enlargement may be due to mucosal hypertrophy or a concha bullosa. Middle turbinate reduction may be indicated to improve access to the middle meatal structures. It may also be necessary for sphenoethmoidal recess and sphenoid ostium exposure.

A conservative reduction of the middle turbinate head may be performed whereby visualization of the middle or superior meatal structures is improved without adversely affecting olfaction, ostial drainage from the anterior ethmoids or frontal sinuses, or the patient's airway (48,49). Care is taken to sharply resect the middle turbinate head while not fracturing or de-epithelializing the vertical lamella of the middle or superior turbinates adjacent to the olfactory cleft. The mucosal membranes on the medial and lateral aspect of the turbinate are also preserved, especially around the "axilla" of the middle turbinate. When a concha bullosa is reduced, a greater portion of the medial lamella is preserved to protect the olfactory cleft.

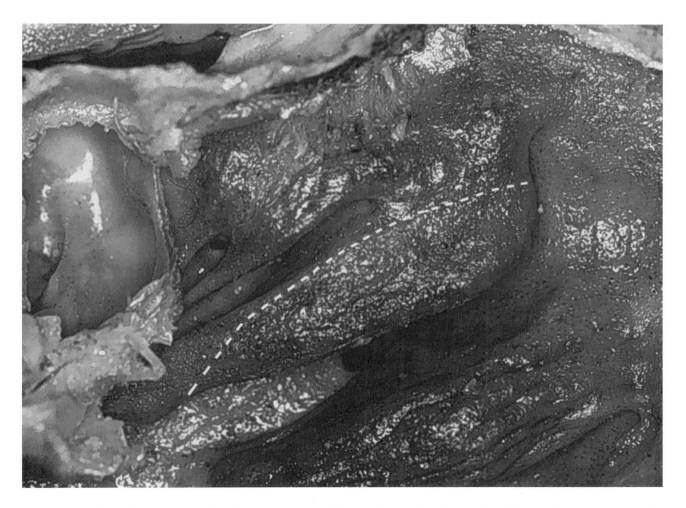

Figure 15 Sagittal view denoting the extent of middle turbinate head resection (dotted line) to expose the middle meatal or sphenoethmoidal recess structures. The vertical lamella of the middle turbinate and the superior turbinate are left undisturbed and unfractured.

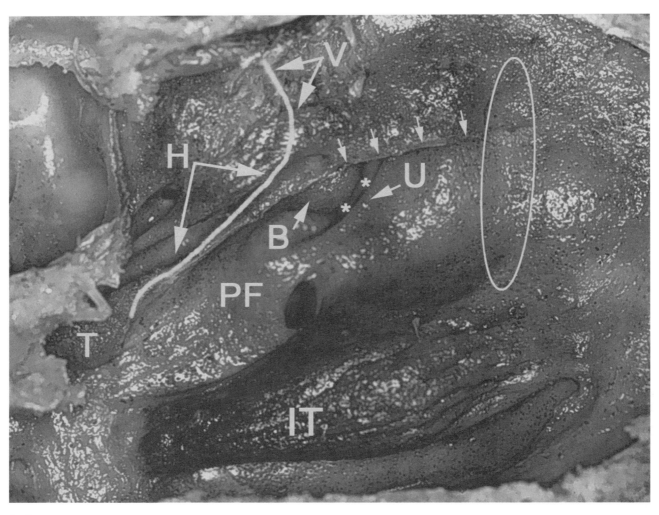

(a)

Figure 16 Sagittal (a) and endoscopic (b) views after middle turbinoplasty. The circle demarcates the nasolacrimal duct convexity in the anterior lateral nasal wall. IT = inferior turbinate. T = tail of the
middle turbinate. B = ethmoid bulla. U = uncinate process. PF = posterior fontanelle with an
accessory maxillary sinus ostium. The solid inverted S-shaped line in the sagittal view denotes
the basal lamella of the middle turbinate as it courses toward the orbital wall. H = horizontal
portion of the basal lamella, where one would typically enter the posterior air cells in distorted
sinus cavities. V = vertical portion of the basal lamella separating the suprabullar air cells from
the superior posterior ethmoid air cells. Small arrows represent the vertical lamella of the middle turbinate.

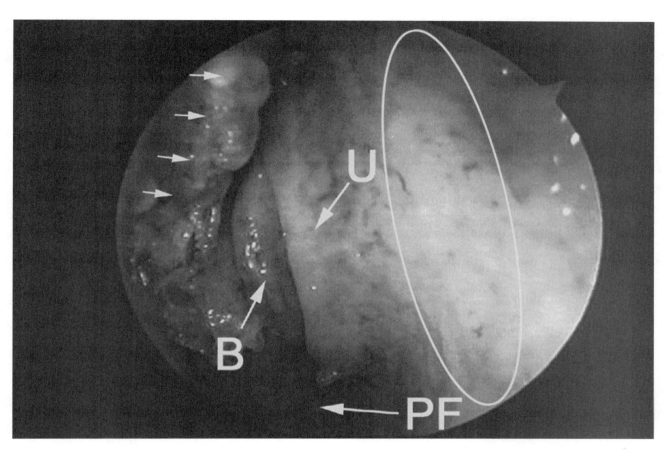

(b)

E. Uncinectomy and Identification of the Maxillary Natural Ostium (Figures 17–19)

Using an angled probem the uncinate process, hiatus semilunaris, and infundibulum are identified. The uncinate process is gently backfractured with an angled probe and carefully removed with a backbiting forceps or powered instrumentation to expose the lateral (orbital) wall of the infundibulum and maxillary sinus natural ostium. Care is taken to conserve the mucosal membranes of the adjacent lateral infundibular wall and ethmoid bulla. In addition, the tail or posteroinferior remnant of the uncinate may occlude the natural ostium. This must be identified and removed in order to see the natural ostium of the maxillary sinus. The superior border of the nat-

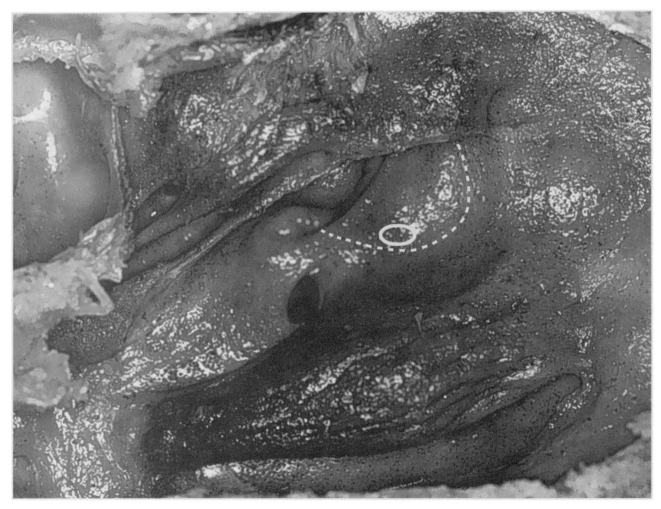

(a)

Figure 17 Sagittal (a) and endoscopic (b) views illustrating the degree of uncinate resection (dotted line) just behind the convexity of the nasolacrimal duct. B = ethmoid bulla. The small circle denotes the approximate location of the maxillary sinus natural ostium behind the uncinate process.

ural ostium demarcates the junction of the medial orbital floor (MOF) with the lamina papyracea. The lateral wall of the infundibulum demarcates the medial orbital wall (inferiorly).

For more limited disease of the ostiomeatal complex, an uncinectomy, exposure of the maxillary natural ostium, and a limited antrostomy may be all that is necessary. However, if there is significant anatomical distortion, then the MOF should be identified through a wide middle meatal antrostomy prior to proceeding with an ethmoidectomy. As the surgeon gains more experience, this step may merely require vizualizing the superior margin of the maxillary sinus natural ostium (representing the anterior MOF), obviating the need for a wider antrostomy.

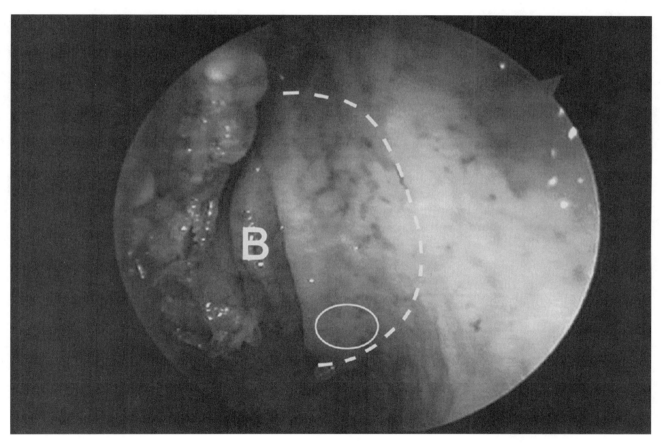

(b)

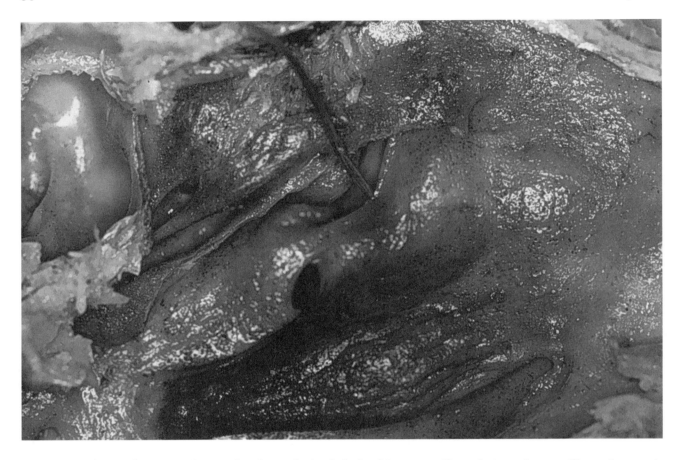

Figure 18 Sagittal view with a probe through the inferior hiatus semilunaris into the maxillary sinus natural ostium.

Figure 19 Sagittal (a) and endoscopic (b) views after uncinate resection, illustrating the maxillary sinus natural ostium (M), the lateral (orbital) wall of the infundibulum (I), ethmoid bulla (B), and posterior fontanelle (PF) area. The uncinate tail occasionally is not completely removed and may lateralize, occluding the maxillary sinus natural ostium and preventing its visualization.

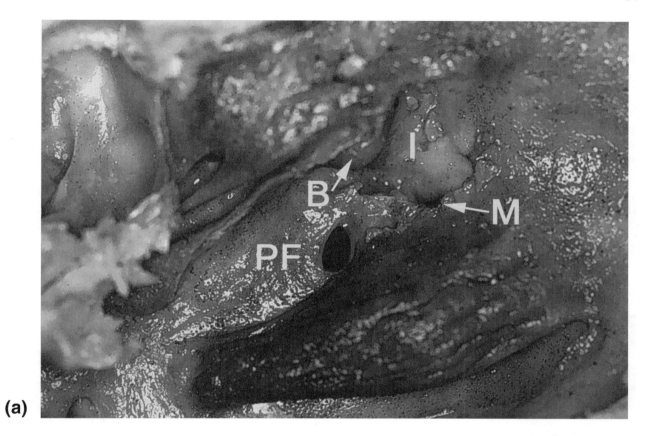

(a)

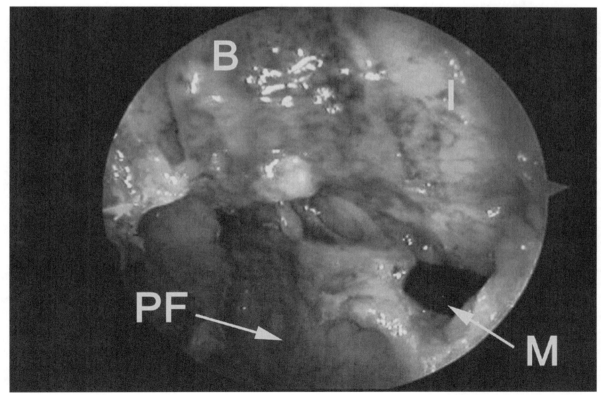

(b)

F.   Middle Meatal Antrostomy (Figures 20–23)

In patients with more advanced disease and/or anatomical distortion due to prior surgery, a wider antrostomy is generally recommended (26–28,37). This immediately identifies the horizontal and vertical bony ridge of the antrostomy, the MOF, and the posterior wall of the maxillary sinus. Combining these three anatomical landmarks with simple-to-use columnellar measurements provides the surgeon with extremely accurate anatomical information that maintains the surgeon's endoscopic orientation as he or she proceeds posteriorly along the ethmoid sinus into the sphenoid sinus. This is especially important in distorted sinus cavities (see Sections G and H below, on anterior and posterior ethmoidectomy). The antrostomy ridge correctly identifies one's location within the ethmoid sinus (i.e., the anterior versus posterior ethmoid cells). The MOF helps in maintaining the correct anteroposterior trajectory as the surgeon proceeds toward the sphenoid sinus. The posterior wall of the maxillary sinus demarcates the relative level of the anterior sphenoid sinus in the coronal plane.

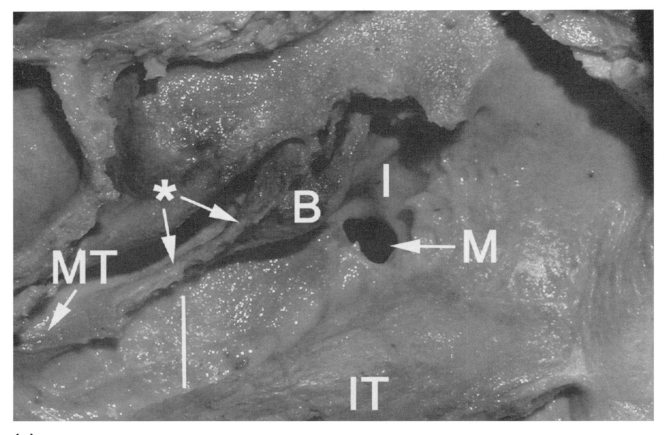

(a)

Figure 20   Sagittal (a) and endoscopic (b) views showing the site of blind entry into the maxillary sinus through the posterior fontanelle area (vertical line). Asterisk = horizontal portion of the middle turbinate basal lamella. MT = tail of middle turbinate. B = bulla. I = lateral (orbital) wall of the infundibulum. M = maxillary sinus natural ostium. IT = inferior turbinate.

In the absence of any "normal" ostiomeatal complex landmarks, or when there is difficulty identifying the natural ostium of the maxillary sinus, the maxillary sinus should be entered through the posterior fontanelle, superior to the posterior one-third of the inferior turbinate. This approach will ensure that the surgeon remains a safe distance from the orbit floor, which rises superiorly at this level. Once the posterior wall of the maxillary sinus and MOF have been identified, by palpation with a probe and endoscopic visualization, a wide antrostomy is created by removing most of the posterior fontanelle and connecting it to the area of the maxillary natural ostium anteriorly.

When performing an antrostomy through the posterior fontanelle area, care must be taken that the nasal, as well as the medial maxillary sinus mucosa, is penetrated. Failure to do so may result in the formation of a maxillary sinus cyst, or mucocele, due to lateral elevation of the medial maxillary sinus mucosa and concomitant disruption of the natural ostium.

The site of the natural ostium is incorporated into the maxillary antrostomy to reduce the chances of circular mucus flow. When the natural ostium is not clearly visible, this is best achieved by removing tissue in a retrograde fashion following the MOF and the horizontal portion of the

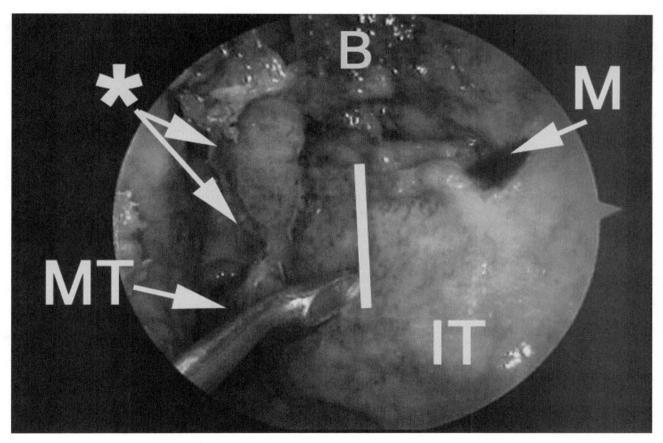

(b)

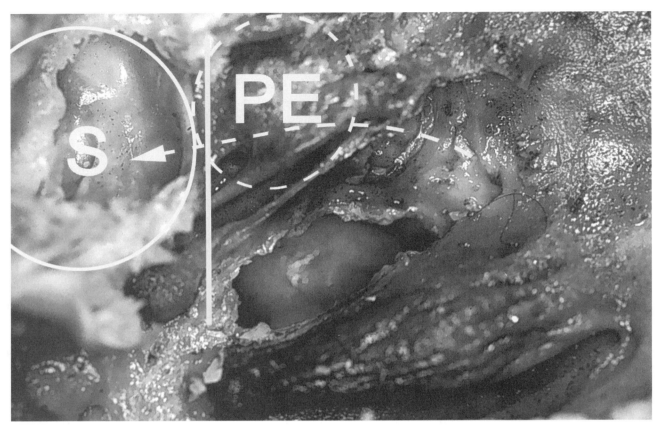

(a)

Figure 21 Sagittal (a) and endoscopic (b) views showing a wide middle meatal antrostomy. The vertical line in the sagittal view denotes the approximate level of the maxillary sinus posterior wall, sphenoid sinus anterior wall, and orbital apex, in the coronal plane. These critical anatomical structures lie approximately 7 cm from the columnellar base. In advanced cases an inferior ethmoidectomy is performed, keeping within 10 mm of the horizontal and vertical antrostomy ridge as one proceeds inferomedially into the sphenoid sinus adjacent to the nasal septum (dotted arrow). S = sphenoid. PE = posterior ethmoid.

antrostomy ridge to a point just behind the convexity of the nasolacrimal duct. At this point the MOF appears to be approximating the lamella of the inferior turbinate.

The MOF and bony ridge of the antrostomy provide the correct anteroposterior trajectory as the surgeon proceeds posteriorly into the posterior ethmoid and sphenoid sinuses. The MOF must always be kept in view and be constantly referred to throughout the surgery. Failure to visualize the superior margin of the antrostomy may cause the surgeon to proceed in a more superior direction toward the skull base.

The camera alignment on the monitor screen must also be periodically checked to ensure that the camera has not been inadvertently rotated. The endonasal anatomy is aligned so that the upper border of the monitor screen corresponds to the superior direction anatomically. The opening of the antrostomy should face medially in the sagittal plane (parallel to the nasal septum), with the

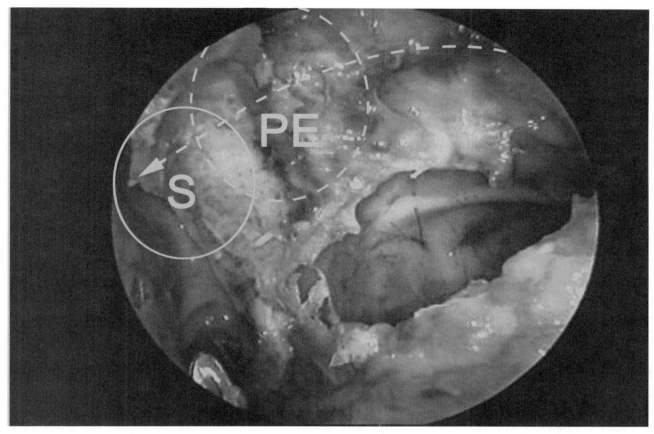

(b)

horizontal portion of the antrostomy ridge and adjacent MOF projecting in an anteroposterior direction toward the orbital apex. The posterior wall of the maxillary sinus as seen through the antrostomy demarcates the approximate level of the anterior wall of the sphenoid sinus, or posterior wall of the posterior ethmoid, in the coronal plane.

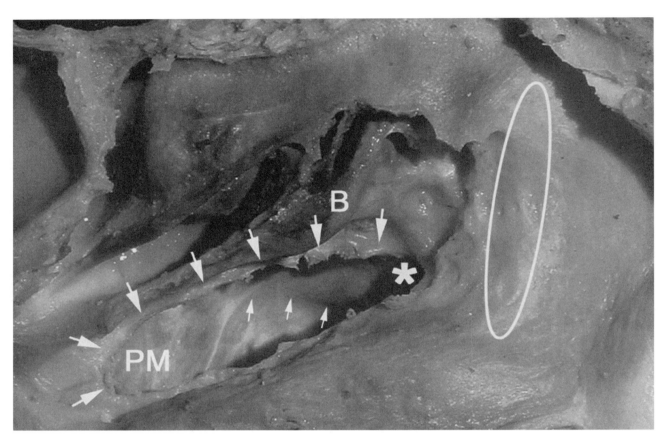

(a)

Figure 22 Sagittal (a) and endoscopic (b) views showing a wide middle meatal antrostomy. The horizontal and vertical ridge of the maxillary antrostomy (arrows) and adjacent MOF correctly identify the surgeon's location within the ethmoid sinus and helps maintain the correct anteroposterior trajectory as he or she proceeds toward the sphenoid sinus. The posterior wall of the maxillary sinus (PM) demarcates the relative level of the anterior wall of the sphenoid sinus in the coronal plane. The asterisk denotes the maxillary sinus natural ostium incorporated into a wide middle meatal antrostomy. Note the location of the maxillary sinus natural ostium adjacent to the MOF and several millimeters behind the convexity of the nasolacrimal duct (oval). B = inferior wall of the ethmoid bulla. Small arrows denote infraorbital nerve coursing along the orbital floor.

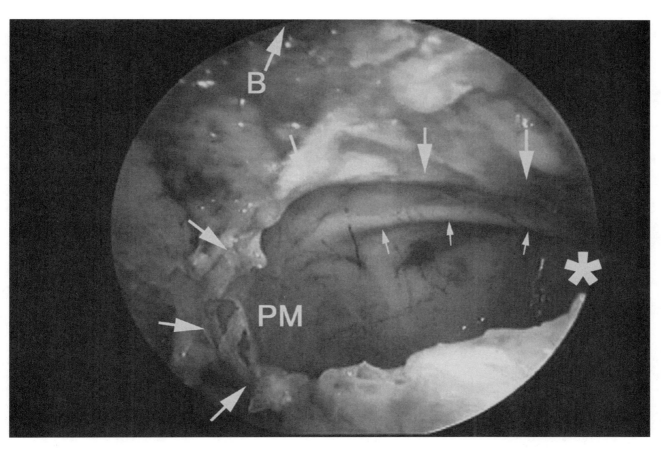

(b)

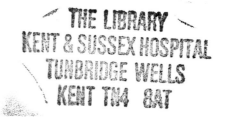

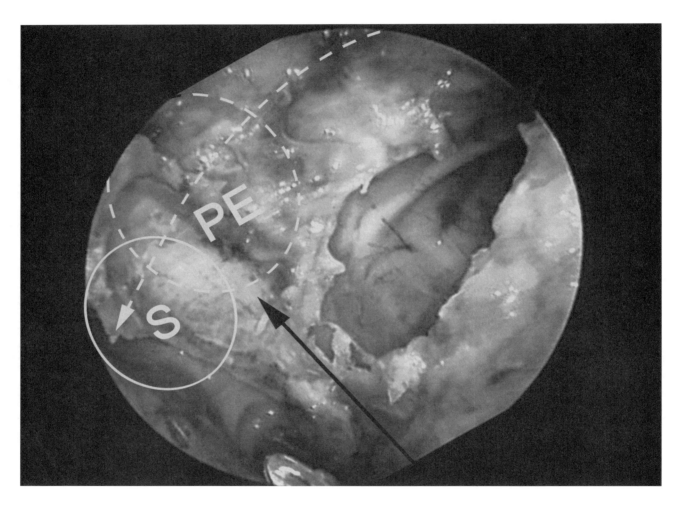

Figure 23 Endoscopic view of improperly aligned camera. The camera is rotated 30 degrees counterclockwise. The solid black line points superiorly. The unsuspecting surgeon may inadvertently penetrate the orbital wall thinking he or she is dissecting "superiorly" into the ethmoid cavity on the monitor. Conversely, the roof of the ethmoid may be penetrated if one incorrectly judges the direction of dissection "medially" on the monitor.

G.   Anterior Ethmoid Air Cells (Figures 24 and 25)

The anterior ethmoid air cells run medial to the horizontal antrostomy ridge. In advanced disease or distorted cavities, the surgeon first performs an inferior ethmoidectomy (anterior and/or posterior, depending on the extent of disease) to identify the medial orbital wall inferiorly (26,37). At this point, the surgeon must begin to regularly palpate the eye prior to exenterating any additional ethmoidal cells. By looking for movement in the orbital wall, bony dehiscence will be identified. A good exercise is to fracture or remove a small piece of bone from the lamina papyracea to illustrate this movement while palpating the eye. The orbital wall, once identified, represents the lateral limits of one's dissection and is followed posteriorly or superiorly as needed (see Sections H and I, on posterior ethmoid and sphenoid dissection).

In advanced disease, the surgeon initially maintains a safe distance of approximately 10 mm as he or she proceeds around the antrostomy ridge (37). This corresponds to the approximate size of a large upbiting forceps. The inferior posterior ethmoid and sphenoid are identified (as described below) prior to dissection of the more superior ethmoid air cells.

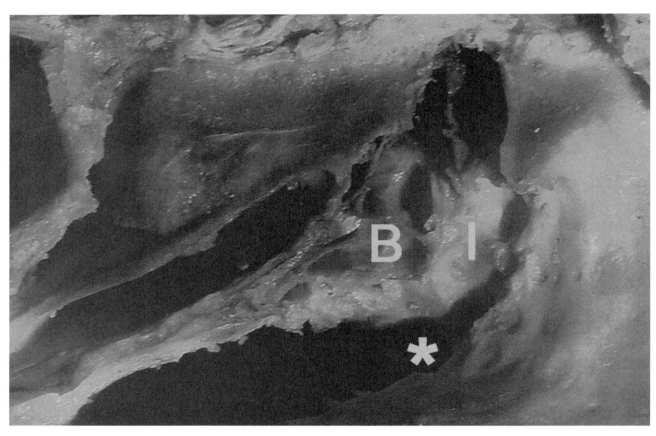

(a)

Figure 24 Sagittal (a) and endoscopic (b) views with ethmoid bulla opened. B = ethmoid bulla. I = lateral infundibular wall. The junction of the medial orbital floor (MOF) with the lamina papyracea makes up the superior margin of the maxillary sinus natural ostium (asterisk).

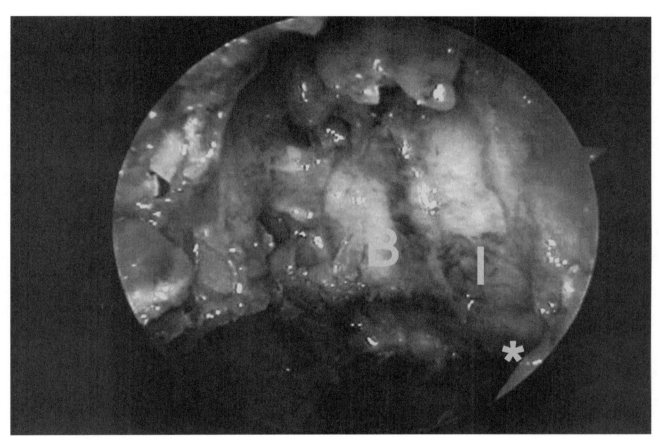

(b)

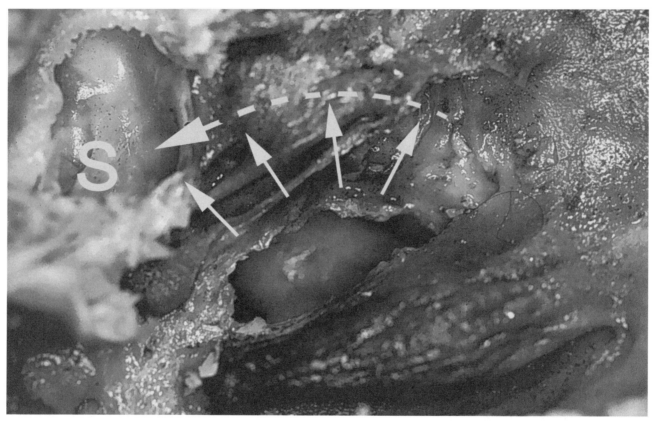

(a)

Figure 25 Sagittal (a) and endoscopic (b) views illustrating an inferior ethmoidectomy. In advanced cases, the surgeon initially maintains a safe distance of approximately 10 mm (solid arrows) as he or she proceeds around the antrostomy ridge (dotted arrow) toward the sphenoid sinus (S).

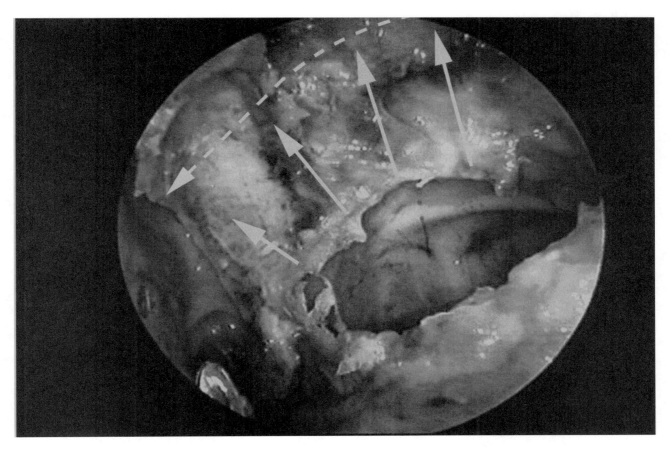

(b)

H. Posterior Ethmoid Air Cells (Figures 26 and 27)

The posterior ethmoid cells may be entered safely through the most horizontal portion of the middle turbinate lamella. Endoscopically visuale an imaginary line perpendicular to the nasal septum from the posterior MOF, another line along the vertical antrostomy ridge, and a third along the free edge of the middle turbinate basal lamella, forming a triangle. The triangle demarcates the zone of safe entry into the inferior aspect of the posterior ethmoid sinus (i.e., through the horizontal portion of the middle turbinate's basal lamella) (37).

Once the lateral (orbital) wall of the posterior ethmoid has been identified, the surgeon may proceed with further dissection of the superior cell(s) of the posterior ethmoid or suprabullar area, thus completing the total ethmoidectomy. The vertical portion of the middle turbinate basal lamella more anterosuperiorly, or other ethmoid septations are carefully removed in a posteroanterior and superoinferior direction. Initially, the surgeon restricts the dissection to an area adjacent to the orbital wall and lateral ethmoid roof where the bone is thickest. Additional passes along the medial ethmoid roof are then performed to open up more medially located cells, once the roof of

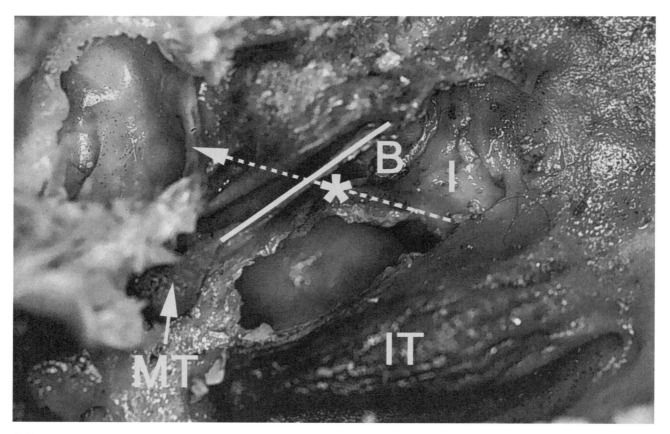

(a)

Figure 26 Sagittal (a) and endoscopic (b) views denoting the triangular zone of safe entry (asterisk) into the inferior posterior ethmoid through the horizontal portion of the basal lamella (solid line). MT = tail of the middle turbinate. B = area of ethmoid bulla. IT = inferior turbinate.

the ethmoid is identified laterally. The surgeon should observe that the roof of the anterior ethmoid roof slopes medially by as much as 45 degrees.

The mucosa along the orbital wall and ethmoid roof is left undisturbed, whenever possible, to avoid granulations, osteitis, prolonged healing, osteoneogenesis, and fibrosis. Only the mucosa overlying the septations is removed. This can be facilitated by the use of cutting forceps or powered instrumentation.

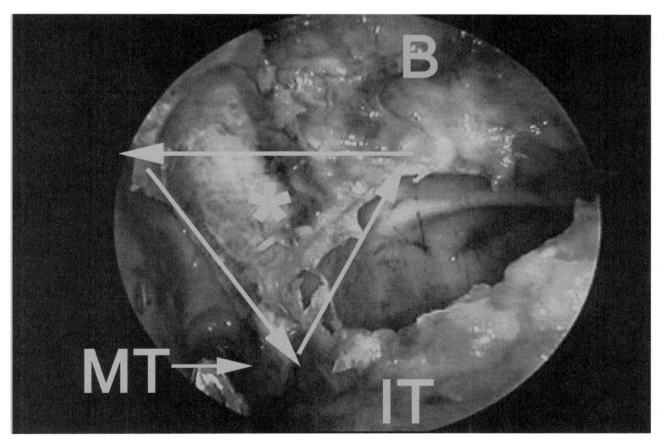

(b)

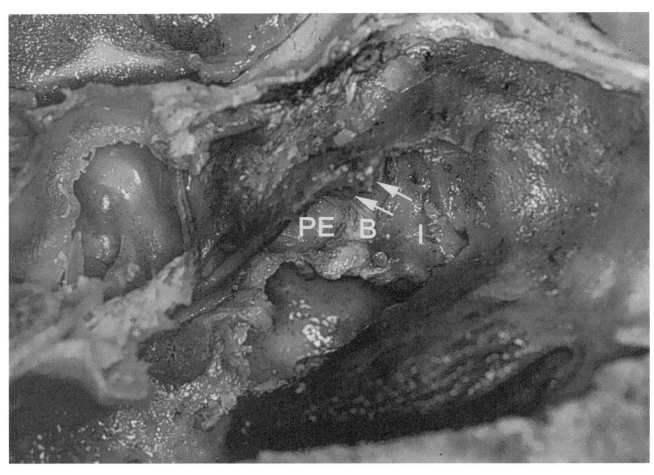

(a)

Figure 27 Sagittal (a) and endoscopic (b) views after removal of the middle turbinate basal lamella. The vertical portion of the basal lamella (arrows) separates the superior aspect of the posterior ethmoid from the suprabullar air cells. PE = posterior ethmoid. B = area of ethmoid bulla.

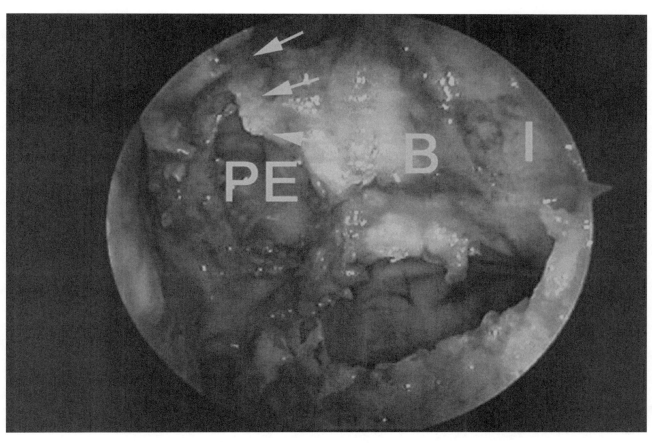

(b)

I.   Sphenoid Sinusotomy (Figures 28–34)

The sphenoid ostium is located medial to the tail of the superior and supreme turbinate and adjacent to the nasal septum, approximately 7 cm from the nasolabial angle of the columnella (37). This area corresponds to the middle third of the sphenoid sinus' vertical height.

A direct sphenoid sinusotomy may be performed without performing an ethmoidectomy or antrostomy. The superior turbinate is exposed endoscopically by reducing the middle turbinate head (as previously described). With a straight ball probe or Cottle periosteal elevator, the surgeon gently palpates the area immediately adjacent to the tail of the superior turbinate and then progresses further superiorly until the sphenoid sinus is entered and the posterior wall is palpated. The posterior wall of sphenoid sinus measures approximately 9 cm from the base of the columnella. The sphenoid is initially opened inferiorly and medially with a sphenoid punch or powered instrumentation. The sphenoid ostium is enlarged laterally only after confirming an air-containing space behind its common wall with the posterior ethmoid sinus. Blind removal, without confirming an air-containing space, can result in inadvertent injury to the intrasphenoidal carotid artery.

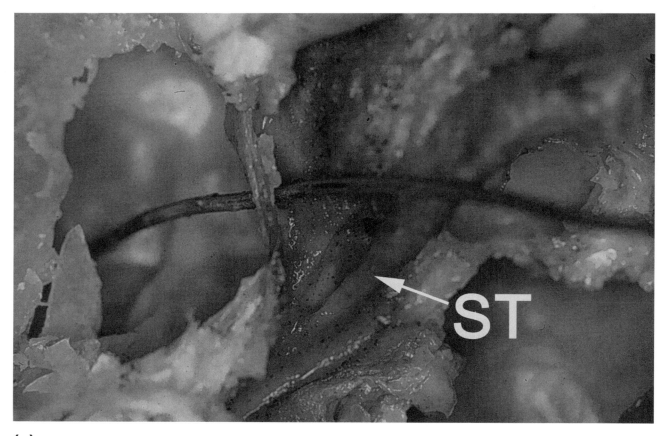

(a)

Figure 28   Sagittal (a) and endoscopic (b) view showing a probe through the natural ostium of the sphenoid sinus (S), which lies adjacent to the nasal septum (NS) and superomedial to the tail of the superior turbinate (ST).

When significant anatomical distortion exists in the area of the sphenoethmoidal recess, and the posterior insertion of the superior turbinate is not clearly visible, then the MOF is used to determine the approach into the sphenoid sinus. In these situations, the sphenoid sinus is entered and identified medially adjacent to the nasal septum, approximately 7 cm from the base of the columnella, at the level of the posterior MOF along the horizontal ridge of the antrostomy. When the posterior MOF is used, the sphenoid sinus will be entered consistently in its inferior to middle third. In most cases, this area also corresponds to the location of the sphenoid ostium. If the maxillary natural ostium (or anterior antrostomy ridge) is used as a reference point, then the sphenoid will be entered slightly more inferiorly, where thicker bone may be encountered. Entering the sphenoid medially, through the area of its natural ostium, obviates the possibility of inadvertent injury to the intrasphenoid carotid artery located more laterally. The latter may occur when a blind transethmoidal entry into the sphenoid sinus, lateral to the tail of the superior turbinate, is performed. Entering the sphenoid medially permits enlargement of the normal sphenoid ostium, thus restoring the normal mucociliary flow of the sphenoid sinus. It also minimizes the chance of creating a separate drainage area through the back wall of the posterior ethmoid sinus.

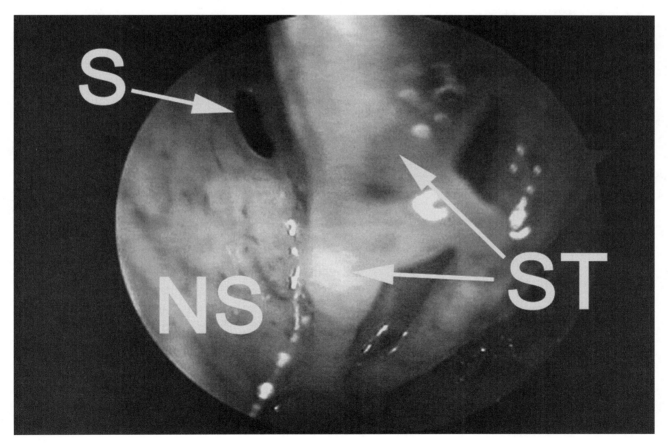

(b)

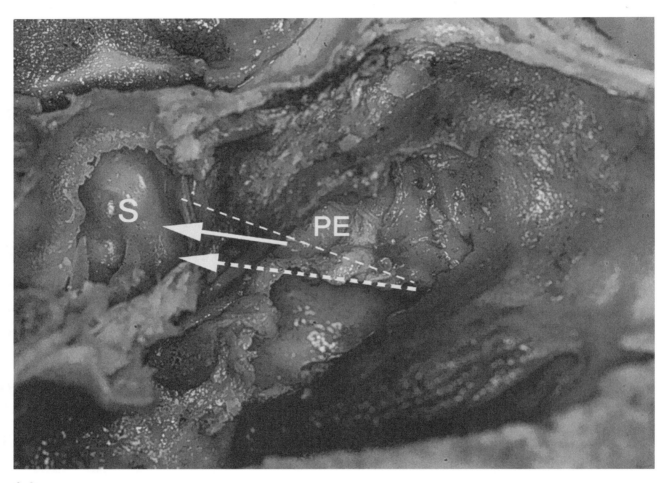

(a)

Figure 29 Sagittal (a) and endoscopic (b) views showing the approximate level of entry into the sphenoid sinus if the posterior MOF (solid arrow) versus the anterior MOF (dotted arrow) are used. Using the posterior MOF will guide the surgeon into the middle third of the sphenoid sinus (S). This corresponds to the area of the sphenoid natural ostium. The anterior MOF or maxillary natural ostium area will guide the surgeon slightly more inferiorly through harder bone, into the inferior third of the sphenoid. The dotted line represents the posterosuperior angulation of the orbital floor toward the orbital apex. PE = posterior ethmoid.

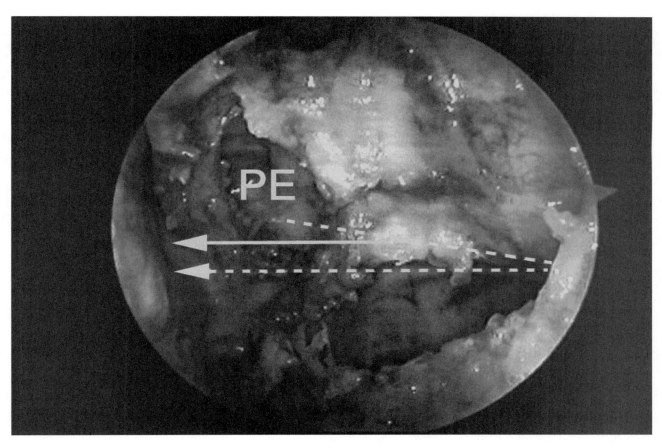

(b)

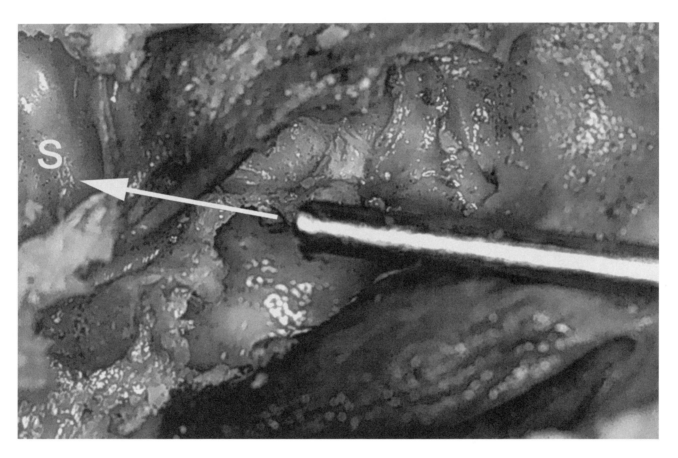

Figure 30   Sagittal view showing the usual trajectory of dissection when the MOF and antrostomy ridge are
kept in view at all times.

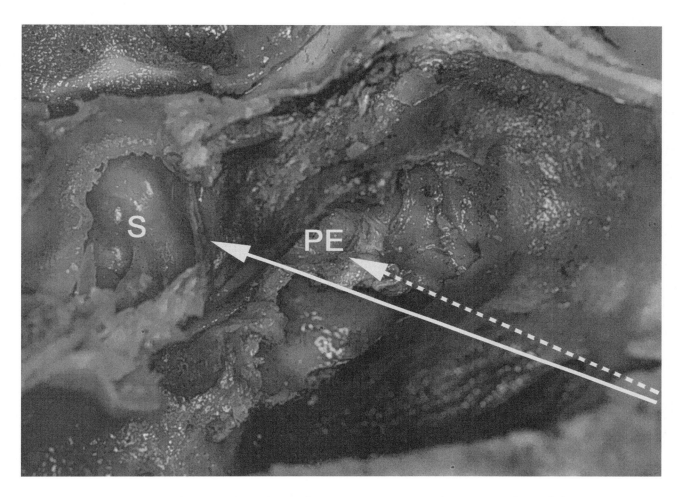

Figure 31 Sagittal view showing the columnellar measurements to the anterior face of the posterior ethmoid (horizontal portion of the middle turbinate basal lamella) at the MOF level (dotted arrow). This measurement is approximately 5 cm. The solid arrow denotes the columnellar measurement to the anterior face of the sphenoid sinus (S) or posterior wall of the posterior ethmoid sinus (PE) at the MOF level. This measurement is generally around 7 cm.

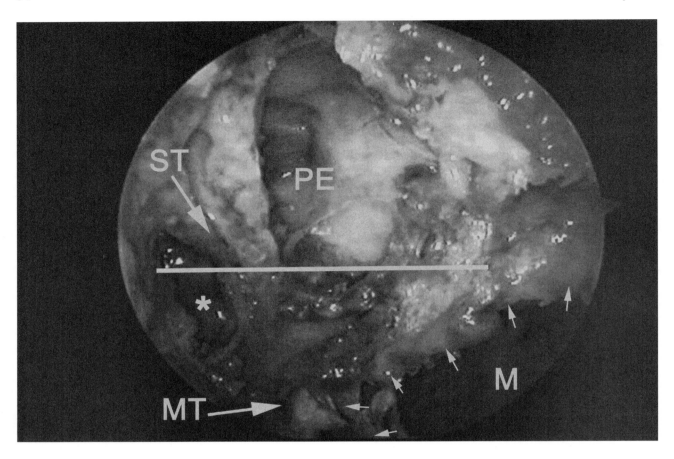

Figure 32 Endoscopic view showing the sphenoid ostium (asterisk), which has been enlarged inferiorly and medially. ST = superior turbinate. MT = middle turbinate. PE = posterior ethmoid. M = maxillary sinus. Arrows denote the antrostomy ridge.

Figure 33 Sagittal (a) and endoscopic (b) views after completion of sphenoethmoidectomy. The sphenoid ostium has also been enlarged medially and inferiorly toward its floor. The common wall between the sphenoid (S) and posterior ethmoid (PE) has been removed. Note the relationship of these cavities to the MOF (arrow). Most of the posterior ethmoid cavity is located above this line. Conversely, most of the sphenoid is located below this line. MT = tail of middle turbinate. B = area of ethmoid bulla. I = infundibular wall.

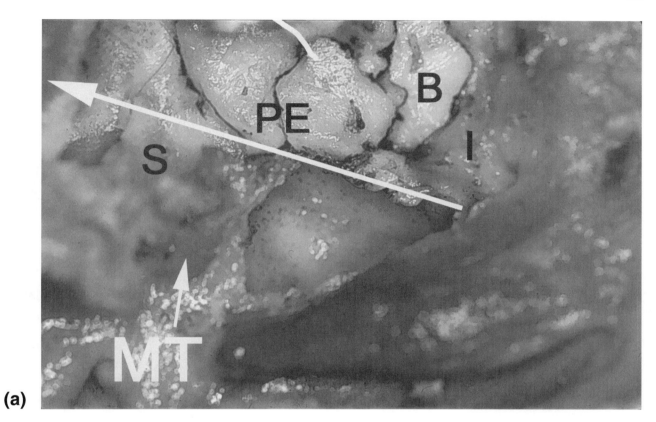

(a)

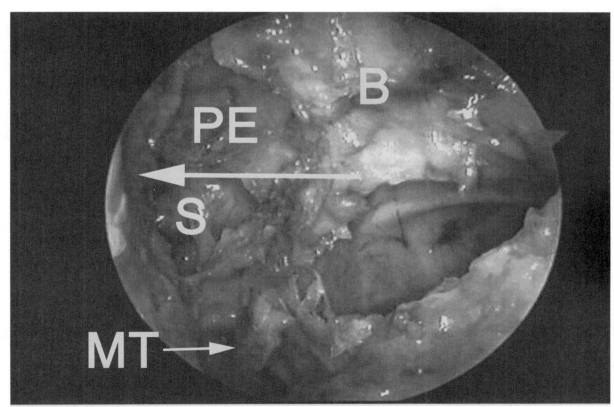

(b)

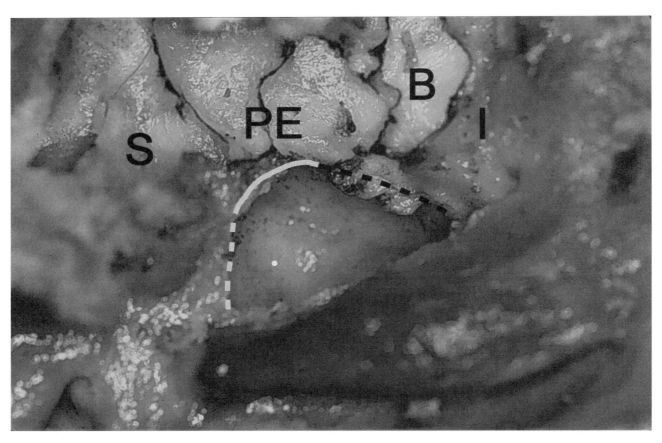

(a)

Figure 34   Sagittal (a) and endoscopic (b) views illustrating the relationship between the horizontal (black
dotted line) and vertical (white dotted line) ridge of the antrostomy and the adjacent anterior
ethmoid or ethmoid (B) and the posterior ethmoid sinus (PE). The transition area (solid white
line) between the horizontal and vertical ridge represents the approximate level where the posterior ethmoid is entered more laterally to this point, through the horizontal portion of the middle turbinate basal lamella.

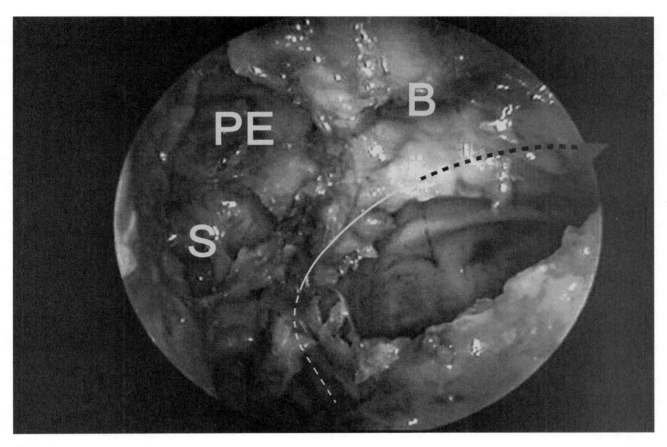

(b)

J. Frontal Sinusotomy (Figures 35 and 36)

The frontal sinus is identified by drawing a line parallel to the bony nasolacrimal duct and directed superiorly from the anterior border of the antrostomy (i.e., natural ostium area) to a point 5 to 10 mm behind the anterior attachment (axilla) of the middle turbinate. The correct point of entry will be directed superomedially away from the wall of the orbit and anteriorly away from the anterior ethmoid artery. The anterior ethmoid artery is located an average of 20 mm (range 17–25 mm) from the anterior attachment of the middle turbinate (50).

Palpation of the frontal sinus' posterior wall is the key to identifying the frontal sinus and opening the frontal sinus ostium. The septations that comprise the roof of the suprabullar cells, and the agger nasi or frontal cells, are gently displaced anteroinferiorly with the angled probe to avoid

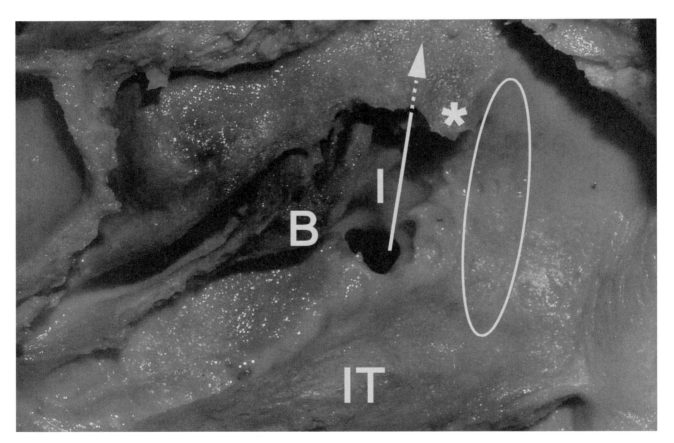

(a)

Figure 35 Sagittal (a) and endoscopic (b) views after uncinectomy and identification of the maxillary natural ostium. The frontal recess is identified by drawing a line (solid arrow) parallel to the bony nasolacrimal duct (oval) and directed superiorly from the natural ostium area to a point 5 to 10 mm behind the anterior attachment of the middle turbinate (asterisk). The correct point of entry will be directed superomedially away from the wall of the orbit and adjacent to the middle turbinate vertical lamella (MT). B = area of the ethmoid bulla. I = lateral wall of the infundibulum. IT = inferior turbinate.

inadvertent penetration into the anterior cranial fossa at the level of the anterior ethmoid artery. An upbiting forceps or giraffe forceps is used to carefully collect the bony fragments. As with the ethmoid, maxillary, and sphenoid sinuses, an attempt is made to preserve as much as possible of the frontal recess and frontal ostium mucosa circumferentially to diminish the chance of prolonged healing, fibrosis, or osteoneogenesis, and subsequent ostial stenosis or complete closure. Through-cut forceps or powered instrumentation with angled cannulas can be used effectively for this purpose. In the presence of osteoneogenesis or fibrosis, more advanced endoscopic procedures may be required (see Section G below).

Transillumination can be used to confirm one's position in the frontal sinus. When the frontal sinus is correctly identified the telescope's light will transilluminate the frontal area. A supraorbital extension of an ethmoid cell will transilluminate in the medial canthal area.

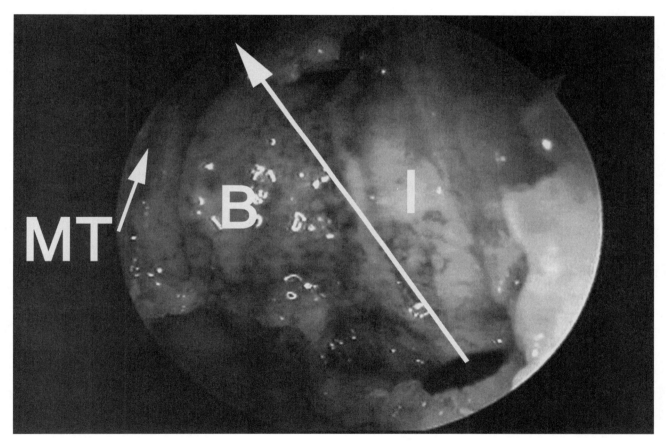

(b)

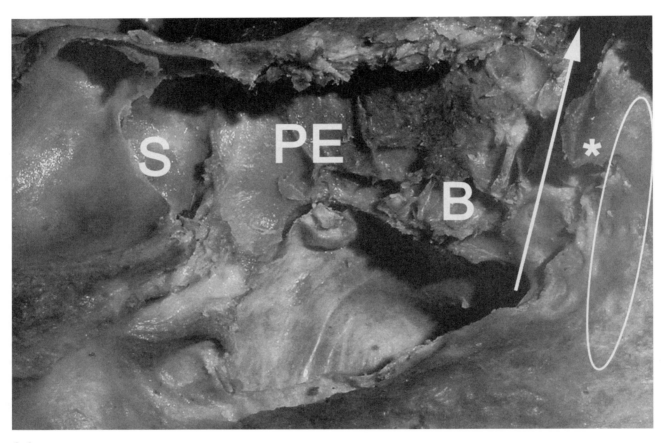

(a)

Figure 36 Sagittal (a) and endoscopic (b) views after completion of total ethmoidectomy and maxillary antrostomy. The frontal sinus is identified by drawing a line (solid arrow) parallel to the bony nasolacrimal duct (oval) and directed superiorly from the anterior border of the antrostomy or maxillary sinus natural ostium area to a point 5 to 10 mm behind the anterior attachment of the middle turbinate (asterisk). The correct point of entry will be directed superomedially away from the wall of the orbit and anteriorly away from the anterior ethmoid artery (AA). S = sphenoid sinus. PE = area of the posterior ethmoid sinus. B = area of the ethmoid bulla. I = infundibular area. M = maxillary sinus. PA = posterior ethmoid artery.

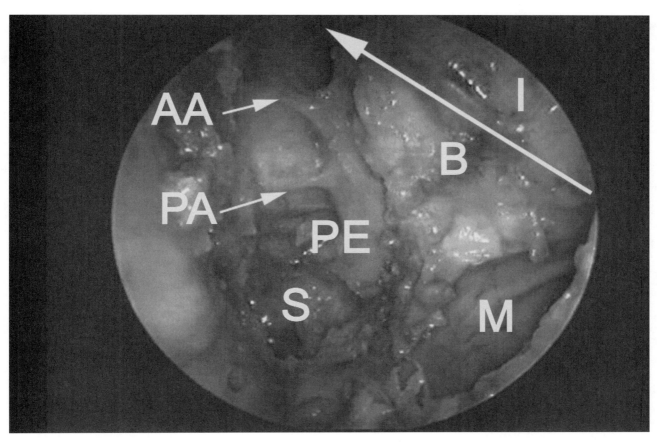

(b)

4

Advanced Dissections

A. Sphenopalatine and Vidian Foramen and Pterygomaxillary Fossa (Figures 37–41)

Identification of the sphenopalatine foramen and pterygomaxillary fossa may be indicated in cases when posterior epistaxis requires endoscopic cauterization or ligation of the sphenopalatine or internal maxillary vessels (51–53). Exposure and control of these vessels may also be necessary during an endoscopic resection of a juvenile angiofibroma or other nasopharyngeal neoplasms (54–57).

The sphenopalatine foramen is circular or oval, and is usually found a few millimeters superior to the tail of the middle turbinate. Occasionally it consists of two separate openings: a larger superior opening, with the neurovascular pedicle supplying the superolateral nasal wall and septum, and a smaller inferior opening, with the neurovascular pedicle supplying the inferolateral nasal wall and inferior turbinate (58). The septal (nasopalatine) neurovascular pedicle can be seen coursing toward the posterior nasal septum and rostrum just inferior to the ostium of the sphenoid sinus and tail of the superior turbinate. Because this branch is often transected in the course of a sphenoid sinusotomy, it requires cauterization. The remaining branches of the sphenopalatine artery supply the lateral nose and anastomose with terminal branches of the labial artery (from the external carotid artery) and the anterior and posterior ethmoid arteries (from the internal carotid artery).

The vidian nerve carries parasympathetic fibers to the nose and paranasal sinuses. The vidian nerve is found coursing along the floor of the lateral sphenoid sinus in a posteroanterior direction.

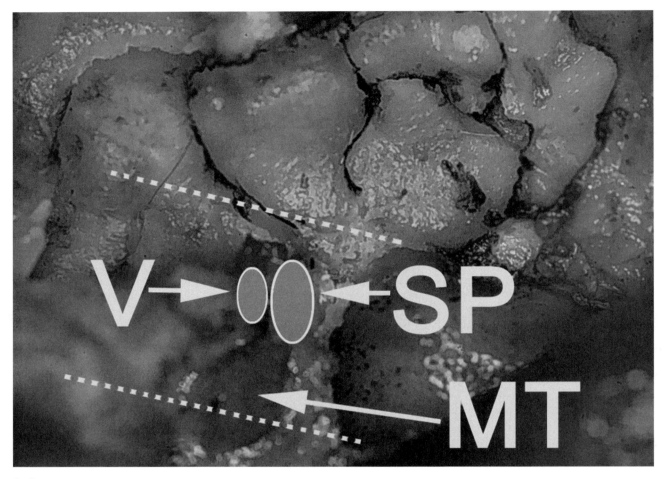

(a)

Figure 37 Sagittal (a) and endoscopic (b) views representing the approximate level of the sphenopalatine (SP) and vidian (V) foramina slightly superior to the insertion of the middle turbinate tail (MT). The sphenopalatine foramen may also be found posteromedial to the vertical antrostomy ridge and approximately half the distance between the posterior MOF and the lamellar insertion of the inferior turbinate into the lateral nasal wall (dotted lines).

The easiest way to visualize the nerve is to expose the sphenopalatine foramen first. A wide sphenoid sinusotomy is then performed to determine the level of the sphenoid floor. The vidian foramen may be found along the inferior bony face of the sphenoid immediately posterior and perpendicular to the sphenopalatine foramen. Nerve fibers enter directly into the pterygomaxillary fossa immediately lateral to the vidian foramen.

The pterygomaxillary fossa can be exposed by removing the vertical ridge of the antrostomy and adjacent thin posterior bony wall of the maxillary sinus through the middle meatal antrostomy. The internal maxillary artery and its branches, the sympathetic and parasympathetic nerve plexus, veins, and buccal fat can be seen within the pterygomaxillary fossa. Superiorly, the infraorbital nerve may be seen coursing toward the foramen rotundum superolateral to the vidian foramen.

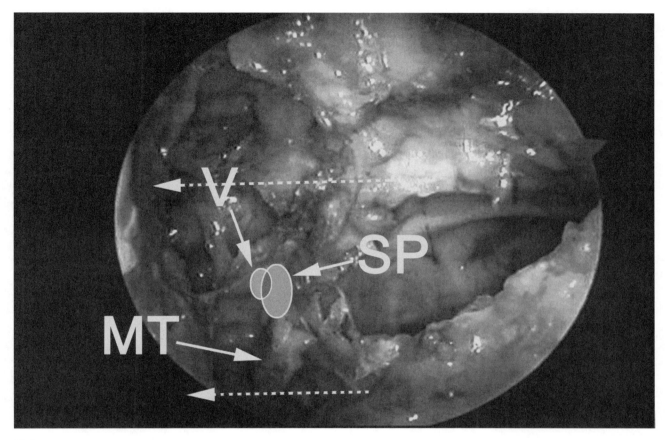

(b)

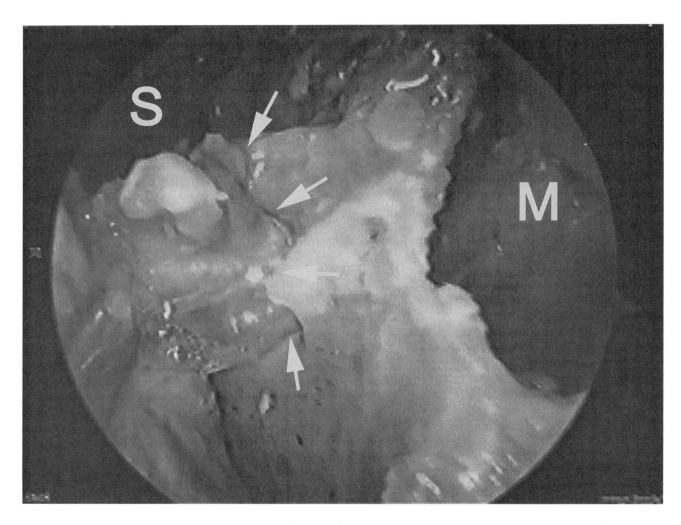

Figure 38 Endoscopic view showing the sphenopalatine foramen (arrows) posteromedial to the vertical antrostomy ridge. S = sphenoid sinus. M= posterior wall of the maxillary sinus.

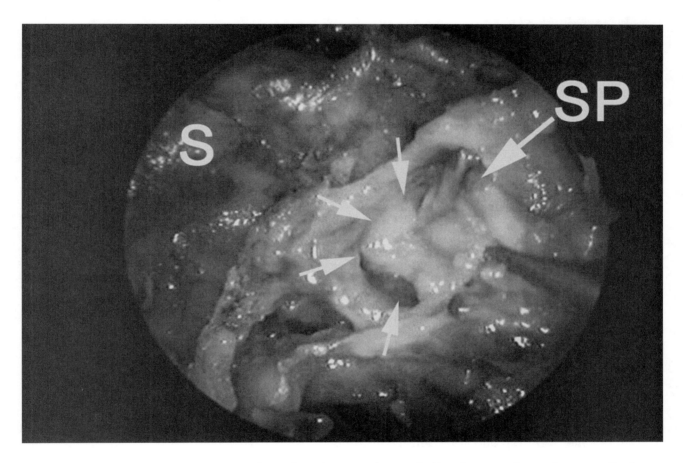

Figure 39 Endoscopic view showing the vidian foramen (arrows) directly posterior and perpendicular to the sphenopalatine foramen (SP). S = sphenoid sinus.

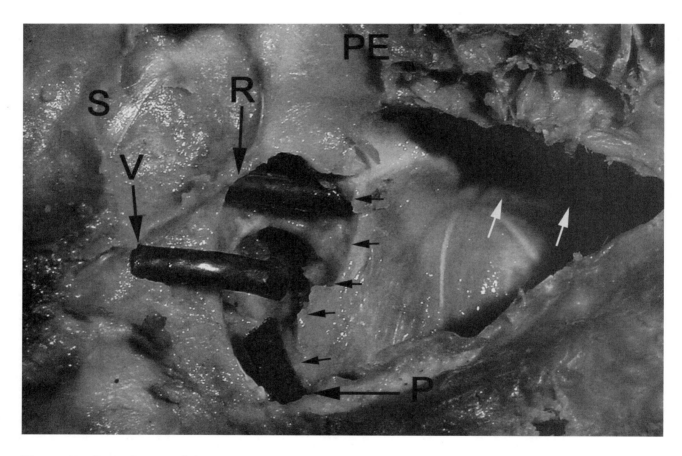

Figure 40 Sagittal view of the pterygomaxillary fossa. The thin bony posterior maxillary sinus wall (small black arrows), buccal fat, and neurovascular plexus have been removed to expose the vidian foramen (V), foramen rotundum (R), pterygopalatine canal, and greater palatine neurovascular pedicle passing to the greater palatine foramen (P). The last is usually found adjacent to the second molar in the hard palate. The course of the vidian, infraorbital, and greater palatine nerves through the pterygopalatine fossa has been marked with black wire. The small white arrows denote the infraorbital nerve. S = sphenoid. PE = posterior ethmoid sinus.

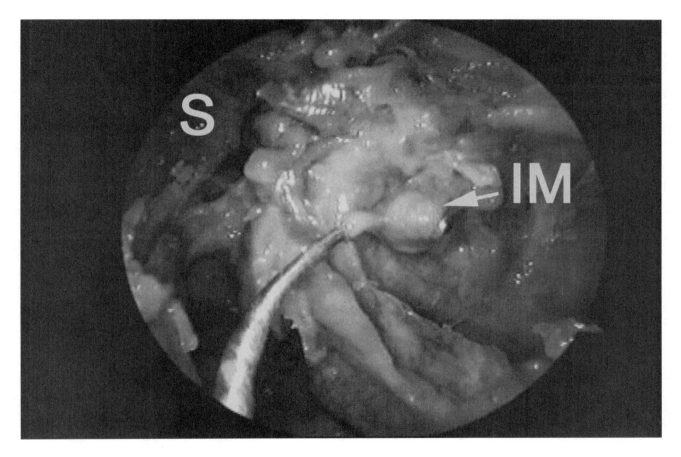

Figure 41 Endoscopic view showing the internal maxillary artery (IM) running superiorly behind the posterior wall of the maxillary sinus in the pterygomaxillary fossa. S = sphenoid sinus.

B.   Anterior and Posterior Ethmoid Arteries (Figure 42)

Endoscopic ligation or cauterization of the anterior ethmoid artery has been advocated in select cases with anterior epistaxis (59,60). The anterior and posterior ethmoid arteries are terminal branches of the internal carotid artery. They can be seen penetrating the periorbita into their respective bony canals coursing through the roof of the ethmoid sinus (50). The anterior and posterior ethmoid arteries re-enter the cranial cavity medially, directly anterior and posterior to the cribriform plate, respectively. Both arteries give off a meningeal branch to the dura as they re-enter intracranially.

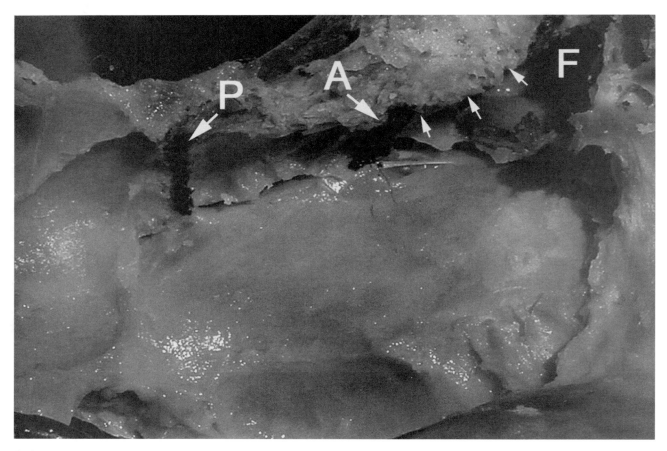

(a)

Figure 42 Sagittal (a) and endoscopic (b) views after removal of the lamina papyracea from the anterior ethmoid area. P = posterior ethmoid artery. A = anterior ethmoid artery. F = frontal sinus ostium. The transition area from the ethmoid roof to the posterior wall of the frontal sinus is seen just anterosuperior to the anterior ethmoid artery (small arrows). Inadvertent intracranial penetration through this wall results in CSF rhinorrhea.

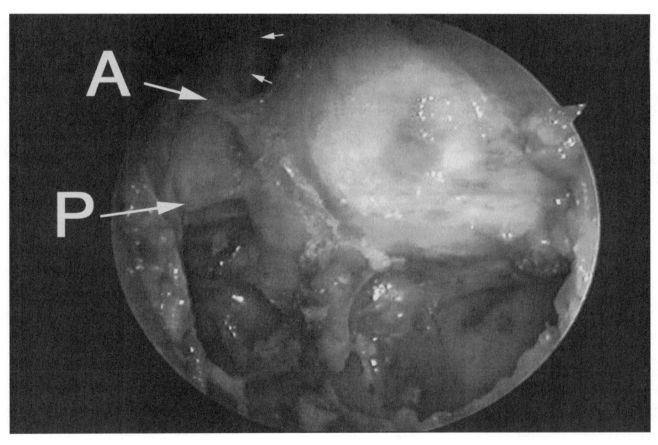

(b)

C. The Nasolacrimal System and Dacryocystorhinostomy (Figures 43–47)

In select cases, an endoscopic dacryocystorhinostomy may be indicated when epiphora is due to nasolacrimal duct obstruction (61–66). The nasolacrimal sac is found anterior to the most anterior attachment of the middle turbinate in the lateral nasal wall (67,68). The nasolacrimal duct courses slightly diagonal and parallel to the uncinate process in a posteroinferior direction toward the inferior meatus. The nasolacrimal duct may be divided into two parts: 1) a bony nasolacrimal duct and 2) a membranous nasolacrimal duct. The bony nasolacrimal duct has a bony wall circumferentially and is typically identified as a prominent convexity in the lateral wall of the nose running adjacent to the anterior middle meatal margin. The bony wall may be very thin posteriorly, adjacent to the uncinate process or maxillary natural ostium. The membranous nasolacrimal duct is located in the inferior meatus and consists of a membranous medial wall and a bony lateral wall.

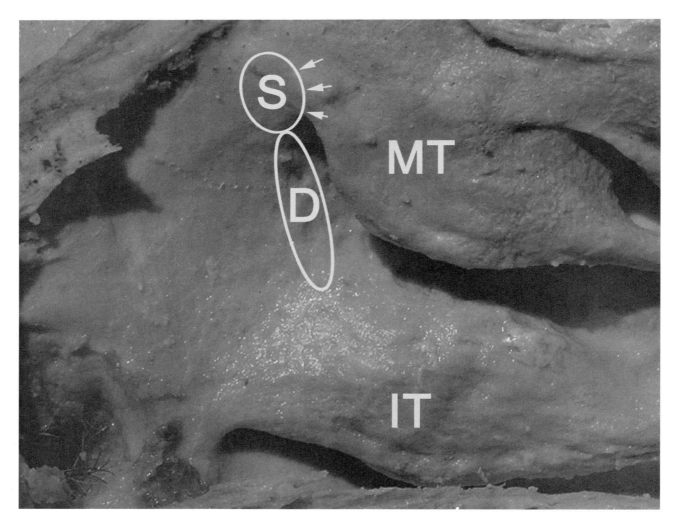

Figure 43 Sagittal view outlining the lacrimal sac (S) and duct (D). Small arrows denote the common wall with the agger nasi cell. MT = middle turbinate. IT = inferior turbinate.

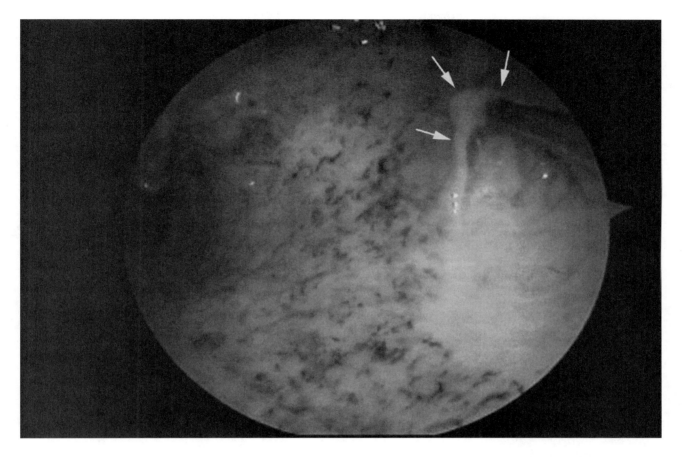

Figure 44 Endoscopic view showing Hasner's valve (small arrows). A membranous canal can be followed superiorly until the edge of Hasner's valve is encountered. A small probe can be used to elevate the membranous wall away from the lateral nasal wall.

The membranous medial wall collapses into the lumen and functions as a one-way valve (Hasner's valve) to minimize retrograde flow of secretions or air into the nasolacrimal duct and sac. Hasner's valve may be seen traversing the inferior meatal wall in its anterior one-third. With a small probe, a mucosal canal can be followed superiorly to identify Hasner's valve and the lacrimal ostium. Occasionally, Hasner's valve is absent. In these cases a patulous opening looking into the bony nasolacrimal duct may be seen in the superior recess of the inferior meatus adjacent to the inferior turbinate lamella.

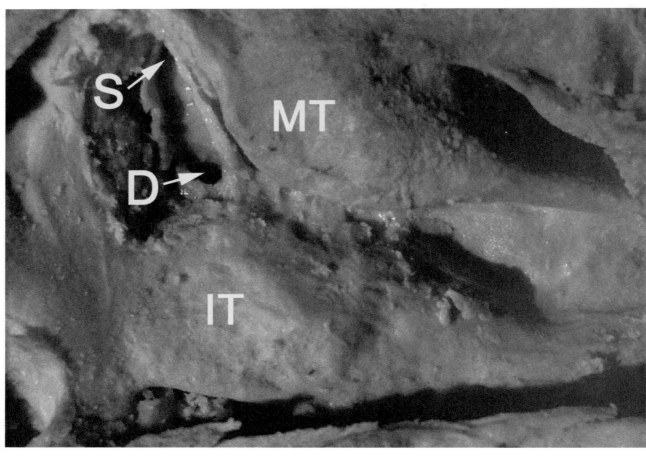

(a)

Figure 45 Sagittal (a) and endoscopic (b) views with the lacrimal sac and duct marsupialized by completely removing the medial bony and membranous wall. S = lacrimal sac. D = lacrimal duct. MT = middle turbinate. IT = inferior turbinate.

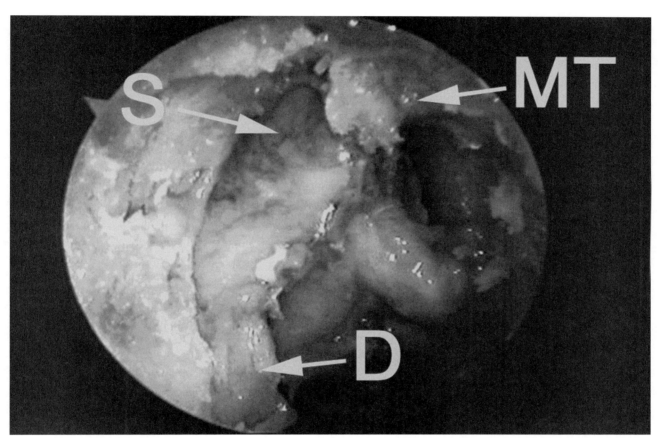

(b)

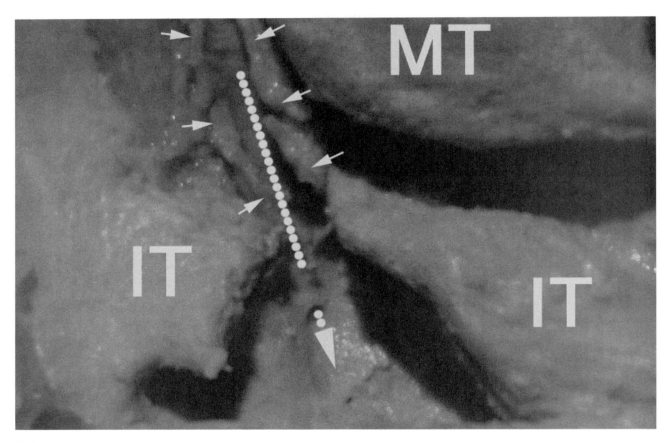

(a)

Figure 46 Sagittal (a) and endoscopic (b) views after removing an anterior segment of inferior turbinate to expose the entire course of the nasolacrimal duct. Small arrows denote the resected edges of the inferior lacrimal sac and duct. Probe illustrates Hasner's valve (H). MT = middle turbinate. IT = inferior turbinate. IM = inferior meatus.

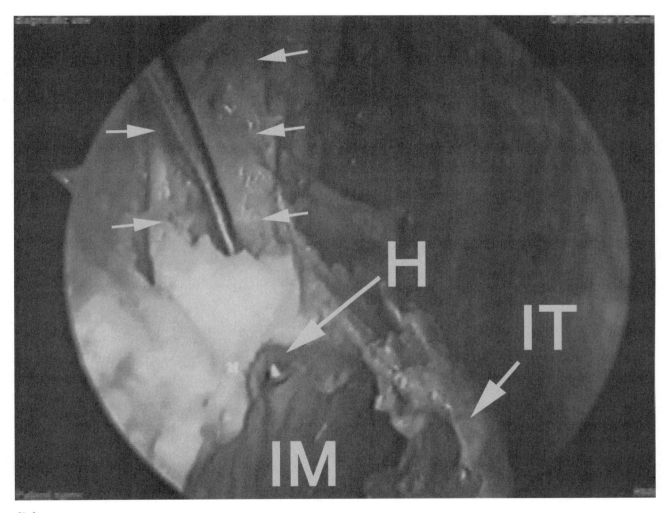

(b)

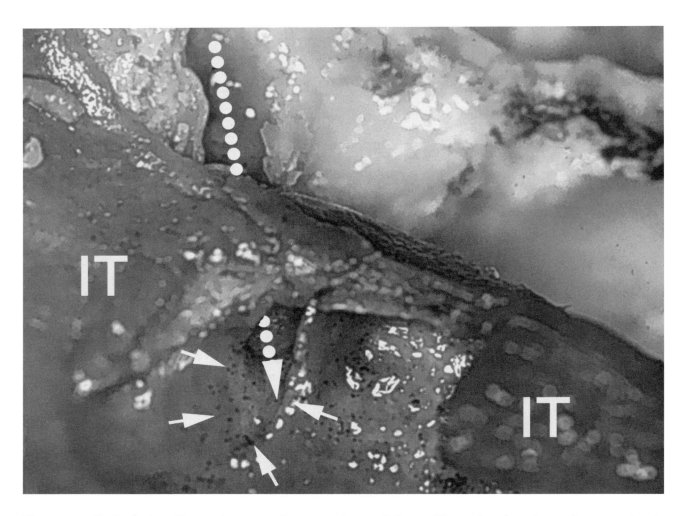

Figure 47 Sagittal view illustrating a patulous opening and absent Hasner's valve. A patulous opening is encountered superiorly in the inferior meatus in some cases. Small arrows illustrate the membranous canal leading up to the nasolacrimal opening. IT = inferior turbinate.

D. Orbital Decompression (Figures 48–50)

Orbital decompression may be indicated for a patient with an orbital abscess, periorbital or orbital hematoma, or severe Graves' ophthalmopathy with exposure keratitis and threatened visual loss (69–79). When a subperiosteal abscess is present, only the lamina papyracea needs partial or complete removal to ensure adequate drainage of the abscess loculations into the nose. This may require exposing the periorbita over the superomedial or inferomedial orbital walls to ensure adequate drainage of all potential abscess loculations. Nasal packing is usually avoided. The periorbita is left intact.

For patients with Graves' ophthalmopathy, the lamina papyracea and MOF are removed medial to the infraorbital nerve through a wide antrostomy. Postoperative diplopia is possible, but may be minimized by preserving the horizontal ridge of the antrostomy (80). The periorbita is incised to allow herniation of orbital fat into the ethmoid and maxillary sinus cavities. The latter generally allows for approximately 4–5 mm of orbital decompression. This may have to be combined with a lateral orbital decompression through an external approach. Care is taken not to occlude the maxillary, frontal, or sphenoid ostia with orbital fat, as this may result in secondary ostial obstruction and rhinosinusitis (81,82). In these situations an extended middle meatal, frontal, and/or sphenoid sinusotomy may be prudent.

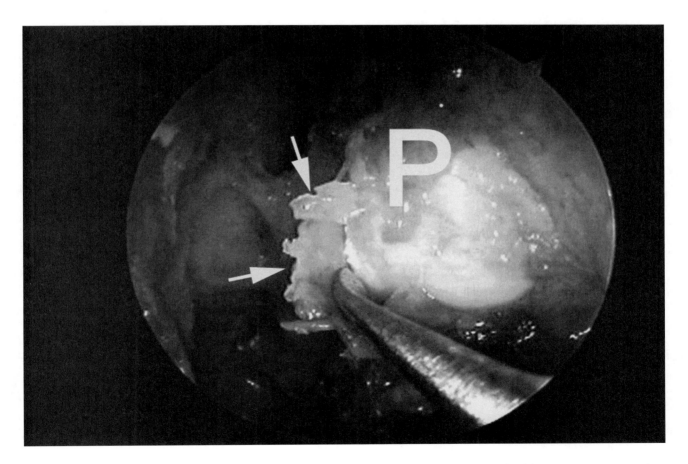

Figure 48   Endoscopic view showing careful elevation and piecemeal removal of lamina papyracea (arrows) away from the periorbita (P). Periorbital abscesses and hematomas occur in this space.

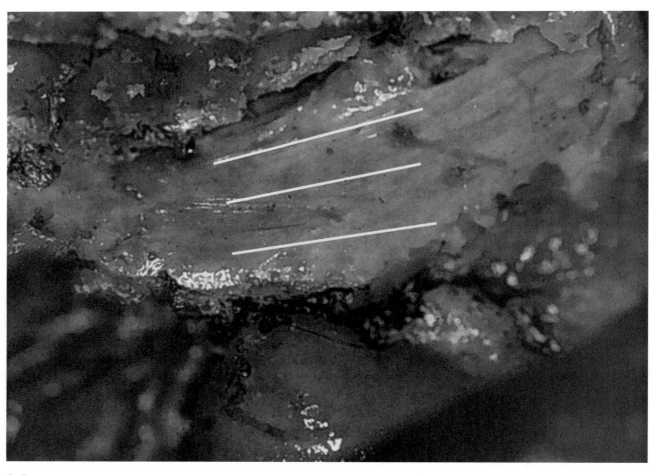

(a)

Figure 49 Sagittal (a) and endoscopic (b) views denoting longitudinal incisions for orbital fat decompression as performed for Graves' ophthalmopathy.

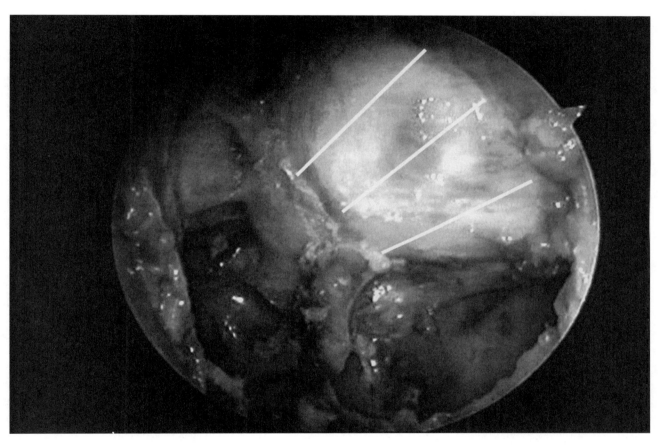

(b)

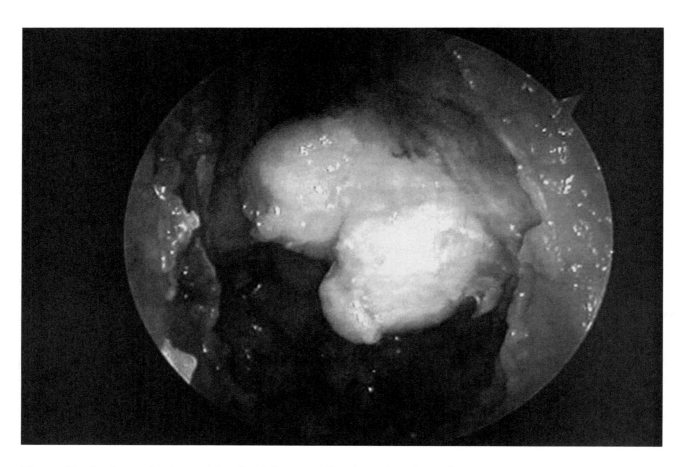

Figure 50 Endoscopic view with orbital fat extending into the ethmoid cavity.

E. Optic Nerve Decompression and the Carotid Artery (Figure 51)

In patients with worsening visual acuity due to traumatic neuropathy or neoplastic compression, an optic nerve decompression may be indicated (83–86). The orbital apex may be found by following a line from the superior vertical ridge of the antrostomy to the roof of the posterior ethmoid sinus adjacent to the orbital wall. It is located at the same level as the posterior wall of the maxillary sinus in the coronal plane, and approximately 7 cm from the columnella. The canalicular portion of the optic nerve is identified as it takes an abrupt turn medially at this point as it courses toward the optic chiasm. The thicker bone in this area is carefully thinned with a diamond bur and removed with a periosteal elevator. In the laboratory this can be carefully performed utilizing a bone curette. The length of the canalicular portion is approximately 8–12 mm. The optic nerve sheath is continuous with the dura mater in this area. Incision of this thick sheath reveals the optic nerve. The space around the nerve is continuous with the subdural space and results in a CSF leak if left open to the nasal cavity. Therefore, if the optic nerve sheath is opened, one must be prepared to close the CSF leak with a small mucoperichondrial graft.

The intrasphenoid carotid artery runs in a posteroinferior to anterosuperior direction, giving it the appearance of an inverted S. Its most anterior (cavernous) segment runs immediately inferior to the canalicular portion of the optic nerve as it courses intracranially, creating a small triangular recess (opticocarotid recess). In some patients with a well-pneumatized sphenoid, the carotid projects into the lumen of the sphenoid and is prone to inadvertent injury if one enters too far laterally through the posterior wall of the posterior ethmoid sinus. For this reason the sphenoid is generally entered medially adjacent to the septum, as previously described.

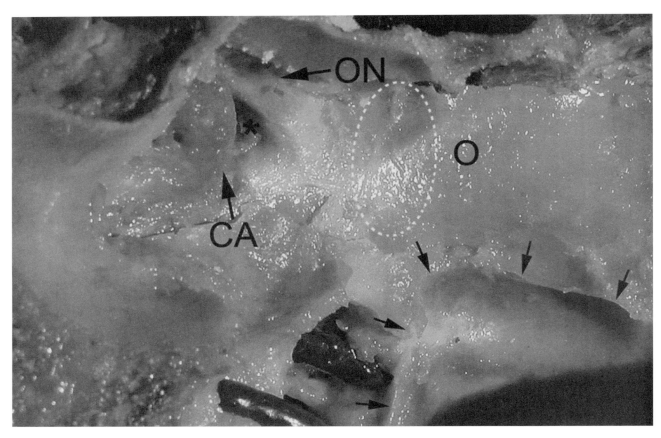

(a)

Figure 51 Sagittal (a) and endoscopic (b) views showing the canalicular portion of the optic nerve (ON) and intrasphenoid carotid artery (CA) after bone removal. Asterisks denotes the opticocarotid recess. The area of the anulus of Zinn (dotted oval) and the antrostomy ridge (small arrows) are shown.

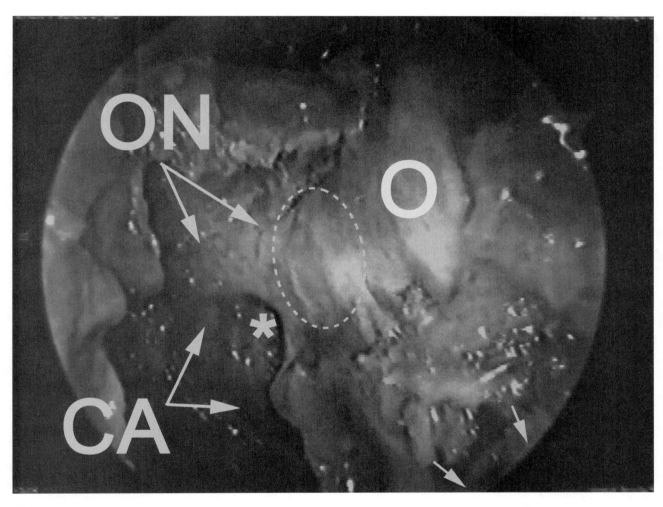

(b)

F. Orbital Dissection (Figures 52 and 53)

Removal of the periorbita and fat reveals the medial rectus muscle coursing along the medial wall of the orbit. The medial aspects of the inferior rectus muscle may be seen running adjacent to the horizontal ridge of the antrostomy. Further removal of fat between the two muscles reveals the orbital segment of the optic nerve and globe. The anulus of Zinn, representing the thick fibrotic insertion point for all the extraocular muscles, can be identified after removing bone at the orbital apex. By longitudinally transecting the anulus of Zinn, between the medial and inferior rectus muscles, one can expose the entire course of the intraorbital and canalicular segments of the optic nerve.

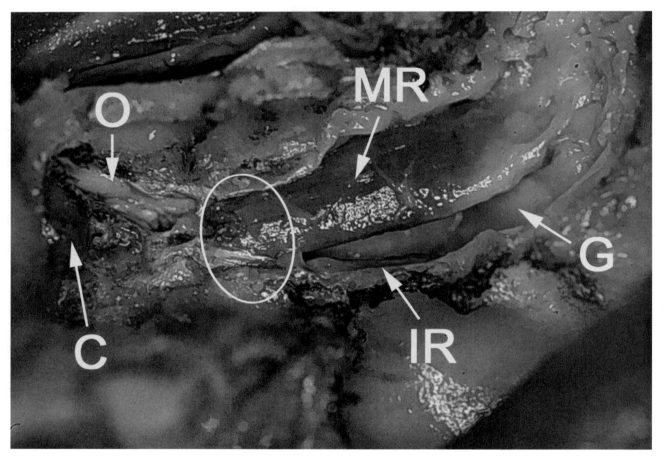

(a)

Figure 52 Sagittal (a) and endoscopic (b) views after removal of the periorbita and fat, showing the medial rectus muscle (MR), inferior rectus muscle (IR), and globe (G). The anulus of Zinn is circled. The optic nerve sheath has been opened to reveal the canalicular portion of the optic nerve (O). C = intrasphenoid carotid artery.

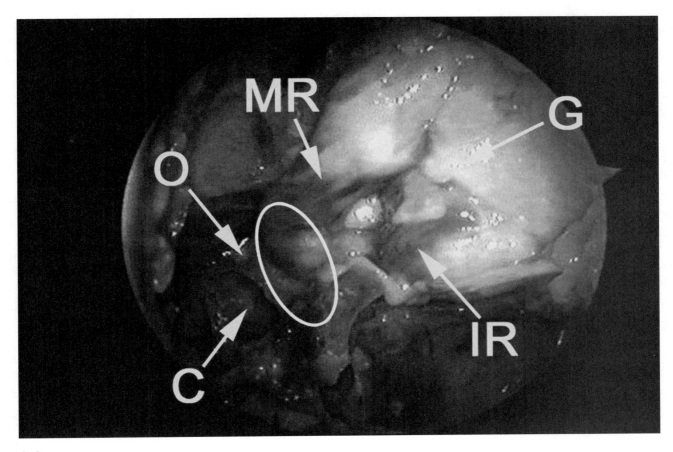

(b)

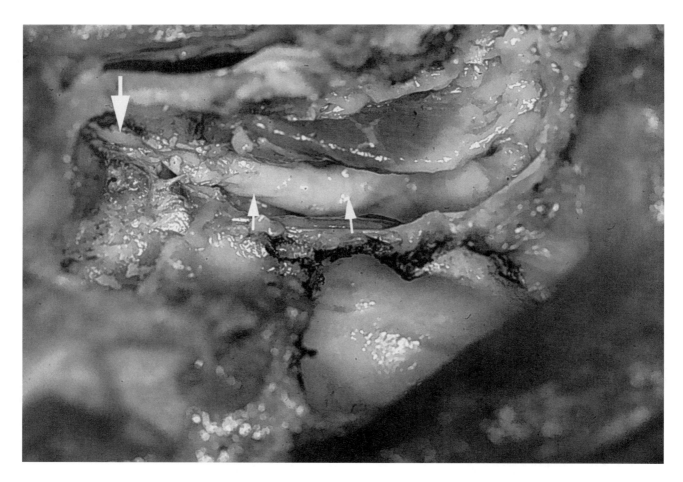

Figure 53 Sagittal view after transection of the anulus of Zinn, revealing the orbital (small arrows) and canalicular (large arrows) segments of the optic nerve.

G. Extended Frontal Sinusotomy and the Lothrop Procedure (Figures 54–57)

An extended frontal sinusotomy may be indicated in select cases with chronic frontal rhino-sinusitis refractory to medical and/or more traditional endoscopic surgical management (87–90). After identifying the superior aspect of the lamina papyracea and anterior ethmoid roof, the approximate coronal level of the posterior frontal sinus wall is determined on at least one side. This may be accomplished either directly through the natural frontal ostium area or through a transeptal approach bypassing this area altogether (91). A 30- or 70-degree telescope looking superiorly is used.

The mucosa on the posterior wall of the frontal recess area is preserved whenever possible. However, in many cases this is not possible because of the significant amount of fibrosis and/or osteoneogenesis in the area. The perpendicular plate of the ethmoid is conservatively resected with cutting forceps anterior to the coronal plane of the posterior wall of the frontal sinus as seen through the frontal sinus ostium or through a transeptal frontal sinusotomy. Posterior to this plane, the potential is increased for inadvertent intracranial penetration, or injury to the cribriform plate and olfactory fibers. An imaginary horizontal line is maintained (in the coronal plane) across the posterior wall of the frontal sinus at all times. The perpendicular plate and intersinus septum of the frontal sinus is followed superiorly, anterior to this line, working simultaneously from both sides of the nose. The perpendicular plate is resected posterior to the nasal bones, and followed superiorly toward the intersinus septum. The dense bone at the nasofrontal area is removed with cervical spine bone curettes, cutting forceps, and/or frontal rasps, until the posterior table of the frontal sinus is clearly visualized. Once the common frontal sinus ostium is visualized, further enlargement can be performed with powered instrumentation.

Occasionally, one or more intersinus cells within the frontal sinus intersinus septum have to be completely removed to create the common frontal ostium. The final common frontal sinusotomy opening is horseshoe-shaped, measuring approximately 8 × 24 mm in the anteroposterior and lateral dimension, respectively (89). The posterior, lateral, and anterior walls of the common ostium are made up of the posterior wall of the frontal sinus, lamina papyracea, and anterior wall of the frontal sinus at the nasion area, respectively. The final ostium should allow for complete trans-illumination and visualization of the full extent of the frontal sinus, including its lateral recesses. If closer examination of the frontal sinus is warranted, a flexible fiberoptic nasopharyngoscope may be inserted through the common frontal ostium.

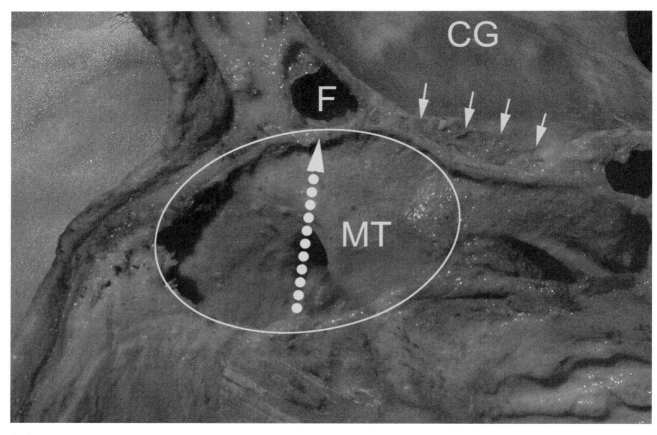

(a)

Figure 54 Sagittal (a) and endoscopic (b) views denoting the degree of perpendicular plate removal (circle) for an endoscopic Lothrop procedure. Care is taken not to extend the septal resection margins too far posteriorly to minimize the chance of inadvertent injury to the olfactory apparatus or intracranial penetration. Small arrows show the area of the olfactory bulb and cribriform plate. A frontal intersinus cell (F) is frequently encountered. The dotted line shows the trajectory for a transeptal penetration into the frontal sinus. CG = crista galli. MT = middle turbinate. NS = nasal septum.

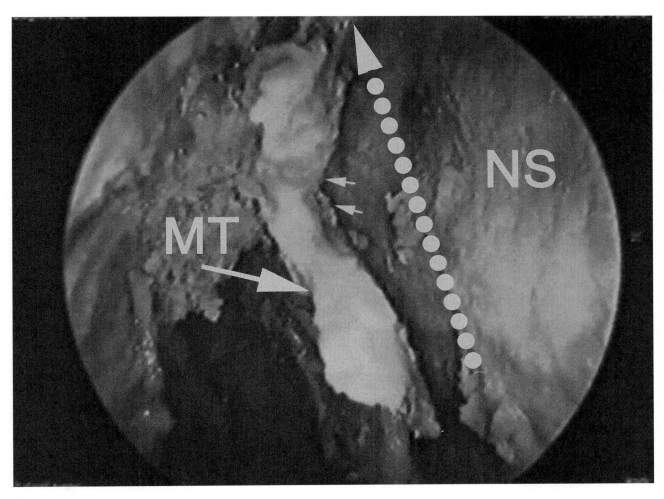

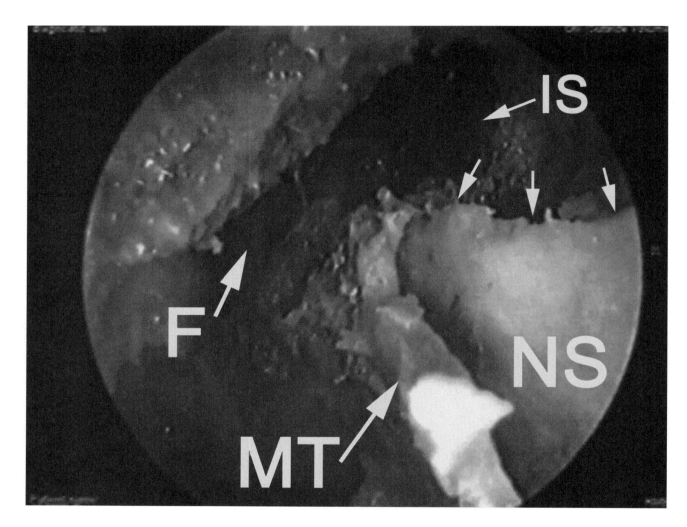

Figure 55 Endoscopic view after medial endoscopic enlargement of the frontal sinus ostium (F). The anterior attachment of the middle turbinate and adjacent perpendicular plate of the superior nasal septum (small arrows) have been removed. The intersinus septum of the frontal sinus (IS) is still intact.

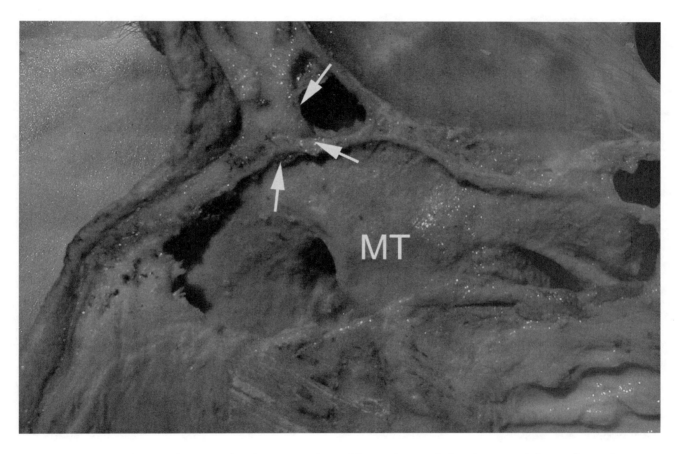

Figure 56 Sagittal view showing the dense nasofrontal bone (arrows) that is removed to enlarge the common frontal sinus ostium anteriorly. MT = middle turbinate.

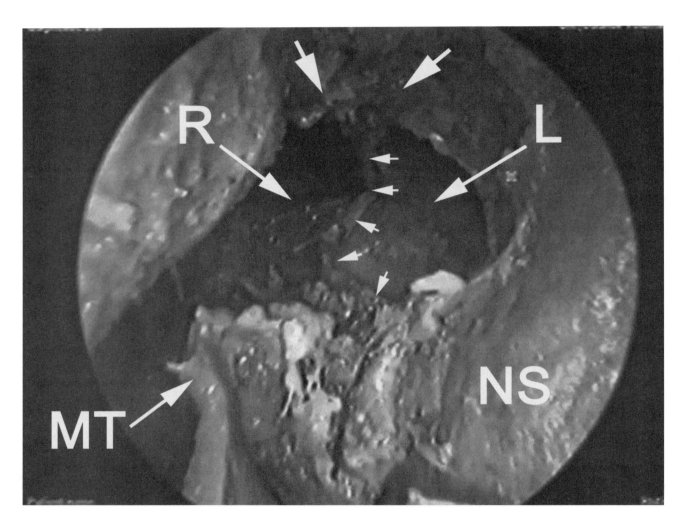

Figure 57 Endoscopic view showing the right (R) and left (L) frontal sinus after removal of the intersinus septum (small arrows). The large arrows illustrate the area of nasofrontal bone needing removal for further anterior enlargement of the common ostium. A left ethmoidectomy has not been performed yet. The latter is typically performed first, bilaterally, prior to the extended frontal procedure. MT = middle turbinate. NS = nasal septum.

H. Extended Maxillary Antrostomy and Medial Maxillectomy (Figures 58 and 59)

An endoscopic medial maxillectomy may be indicated for patients with a variety of benign and malignant nasal and paranasal sinus neoplasms. Perhaps the most common indication, however, is for the resection of inverted papillomas (92–97). The resection begins with a complete inferior turbinectomy. The medial maxillary wall is then resected, beginning with a maxillary antrostomy at the inferior meatus as described previously. The margins of resection for the medial maxillectomy are: 1) the floor of the nose inferiorly, 2) the posterior wall of the maxillary sinus posteriorly, 3) the floor of the orbit superiorly, and 4) the anterior maxillary wall anteriorly. The last requires resection of the osseus and membranous nasolacrimal duct. The procedure then proceeds with an anterior ethmoidectomy, posterior ethmoidectomy, and wide sphenoidotomy with complete removal of the mucous membranes if involved by neoplasm. The thin lamina papyracea and adjacent MOF are carefully removed from the anterior and posterior ethmoid cavity with a periosteal

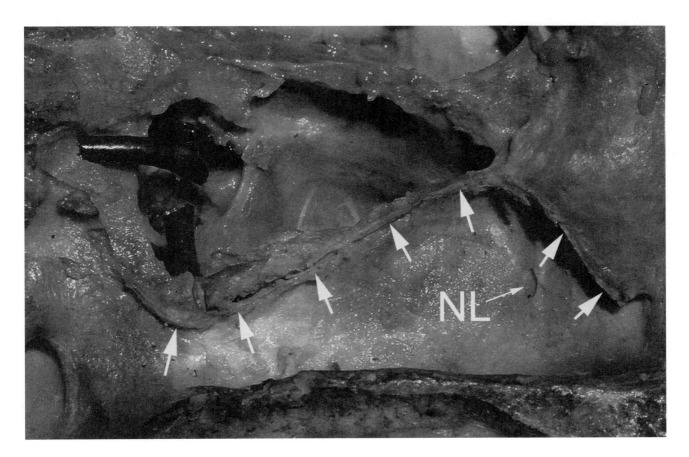

Figure 58 Sagittal view after complete removal of the inferior turbinate, including the lamellar attachment to the lateral wall (arrows). The entire medial maxillary wall is removed flush with the anterior and posterior maxillary sinus wall, orbital floor, and nasal floor. The nasolacrimal duct is usually removed to expose the anterior maxillary sinus wall. Also, a total ethmoidectomy and removal of the lamina papyracea are typically performed as part of a medial maxillectomy. NL = Hasner's valve and membranous lacrimal duct in the inferior meatus. Note the mucosal canal denoting the location of Hasner's valve.

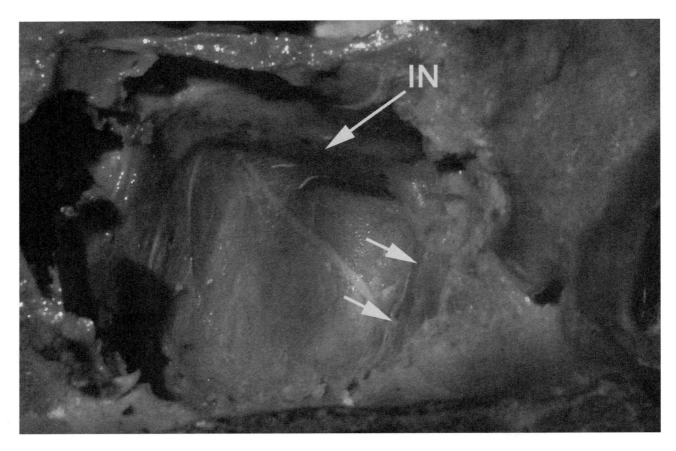

Figure 59 Sagittal view after complete medial maxillary sinus wall removal. IN = infraorbital nerve and vessels. Arrows show the anterior maxillary sinus wall after removal of the nasolacrimal duct.

elevator. The thickest bone will be encountered anteriorly at the nasolacrimal duct, inferiorly along the horizontal ridge of the antrostomy, posteriorly at the orbital apex, and superiorly at the junction of the ethmoid roof and orbital wall. Therefore, it may be necessary to thin these areas of thick bone with a burr prior to removal with a periosteal elevator. A dacryocystorhinostomy is performed at the end of the procedure to minimize the chance of nasolacrimal sac stenosis or closure. Tissue samples from the various sinus cavities or turbinates are sent in separate tissue containers for pathological evaluation and for subsequent postoperative pathological mapping of the various cavities and nasal structures. This postoperative pathological map is used to illustrate which sinuses are involved with neoplasm versus inflammatory disease. It can also be used to guide further treatment if indicated, e.g., radiation therapy or further radical external surgery.

Patients with more extensive involvement of the frontal sinus may require an endoscopic Lothrop procedure to improve exposure of the frontal sinus cavity and to facilitate the postoperative management and evaluation of these cavities for recurrence. If disease appears to involve the ethmoid roof, a medium-sized otologic diamond burr on an angled handpiece is used to thin it down. Although generally not necessary in most cases, bone removal from the ethmoid roof can be completed in a piecemeal fashion with a periosteal elevator. More extensive bilateral disease involving the septum or sphenoid sinus may require a septectomy and/or an extended sphenoid sinusotomy with removal of the sphenoid rostrum and intersinus septum.

I. Extended Sphenoid Sinusotomy and Approach to the Sella Turcica
(Figures 60 and 61)

Endoscopic resection of pituitary adenomas has been reported (98–102). In these cases, an extended sphenoid sinusotomy is necessary to gain exposure to the sella turcica. In addition, an extended sphenoid sinusotomy may be necessary to improve access to a lateral sphenoid recess behind the medial pterygomaxillary fossa, to improve visualization while repairing a CSF leak, or for exposure and removal of a meningoencephalocele (103–105). The approach to the pituitary fossa begins with an extended sphenoid sinusotomy. The sphenoid sinus is initially opened bilaterally, as previously mentioned. The rostrum and intersinus septum are sharply resected with bone-cutting forceps or powered instrumentation. Occasionally the intersinus septum may attach to the anterior wall of the carotid artery. For this reason care is taken to avoid fracturing or inadvertently pulling the intersinus septum to prevent tearing the carotid. In a well-pneumatized sphenoid sinus, the pituitary fossa will often be seen as a convexity in the roof of the common sphenoid cavity (106). However, the surgeon localizes the fossa with intraoperative fluoroscopy or another intraoperative imaging device prior to bone removal. Once the pituitary fossa is localized, the

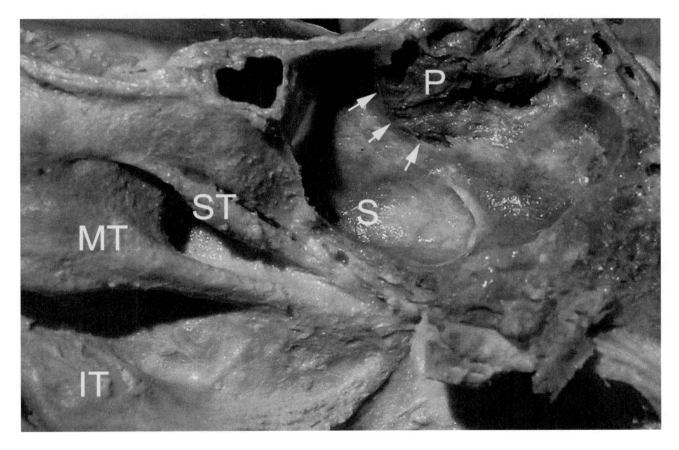

Figure 60   Sagittal view. IT = inferior turbinate. MT = middle turbinate. ST = superior turbinate. S = sphenoid. In a well-pneumatized sphenoid sinus, the pituitary fossa (P) will often be seen as a convexity (arrows) in the roof of the common sphenoid cavity.

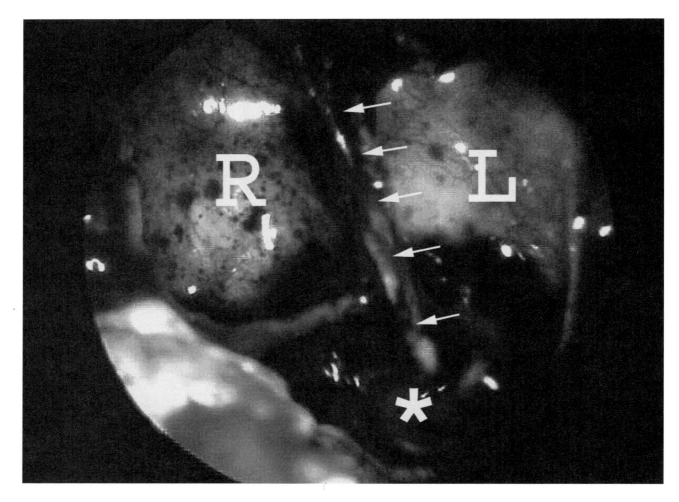

Figure 61   Endoscopic view. R = right sphenoid sinus. L = left sphenoid sinus. Small arrows denoted the resected edge of the sphenoid intersinus septum. An intersinus (rostrum) air cell is seen inferiorly (asterisk).

bone is thinned with a cutting or diamond burr and the bone is gently removed to expose the capsule of the pituitary gland. The capsule is then incised, exposing the pituitary gland or neoplasm within the sella turcica.

J. Anterior Skull-Base Resection (Figure 62)

Endoscopic resection of anterior skull-base neoplasms may be used as an adjunct to traditional (endoscopic-assisted) external approaches (107,108). It may also be performed as the only procedure in select cases, obviating the need for external incisions or a frontal craniotomy (109). Preoperative computer tomography and magnetic resonance imaging are useful in differentiating neoplasm from inflammatory disease, and for the preoperative surgical planning in all these cases.

The intranasal component of the neoplasm is debulked, as in an extensive nasal polyposis case, to expose the nasal septum, lateral nasal wall, and posterior choanal structures. The remaining parts of the procedure are performed principally with noncutting forceps to ensure adequate mucosal stripping and to yield tissue for final pathological analysis and postoperative mapping of the involved areas. A suction filter (sock) is used to collect the tissue debris if powered dissection is used. If bilateral surgery is performed, one sock is used for each side and labeled appropriately for pathological analysis.

An endoscopic medial maxillectomy is performed if the tumor appears to involve the ethmoid sinus. A total ethmoidectomy and a middle meatal antrostomy are also performed on the con-

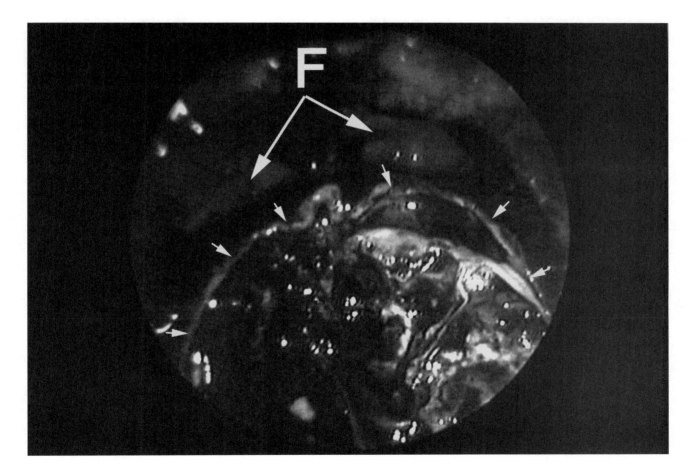

Figure 62 Endoscopic resection of an anterior skull base lesion. F = common frontal ostium after an endoscopic Lothrop procedure. Arrows denote resected dural margins from orbit to orbit.

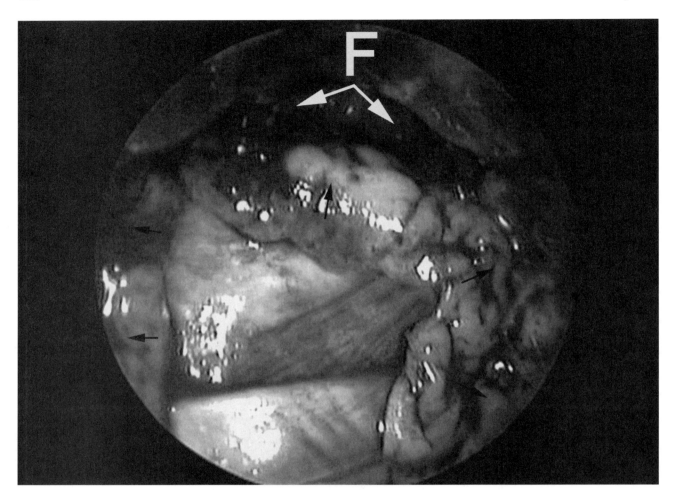

Figure 63 Repair of a large 3 × 2 cm anterior skull base defect with lyophilized dura and mucosal grafts. F = common frontal sinus ostium after a Lothrop procedure.

tralateral side if tumor appears to extend beyond the confines of the ipsilateral olfactory cleft and the adjacent perpendicular plate of the nasal septum and/or crista galli. The nasal septum is removed back to uninvolved margins, allowing the surgeon to operate through both nares simultaneously. A contralateral secondary suction is used to continuously clear the nasopharynx of blood and debris. The sphenopalatine foramen is identified and cauterized bilaterally.

The skull-base resection starts with an extended frontal sinusotomy (the Lothrop procedure), as described previously. This allows exposure of the anterior margins of resection and removal of involved soft tissues at the nasoseptal angle just posterior to the nasion and nasal bones. Large (6–12-mm) cutting burrs are used to thin involved bone at the nasofrontal suture line (nasion) and to widely expand the common frontal sinusotomy, exposing the posterior table of the frontal sinus (as previously described). An extended sphenoid sinusotomy is performed by removing the remaining rostrum and intersinus septum of the sphenoid sinus along with the mucosa. The optic nerves and carotid arteries are identified bilaterally. The bony ethmoid and sphenoid roof anterior to the optic chiasm are thinned with large cutting burrs to eggshell thickness and removed to expose the underlying dura circumferentially (around the remaining perpendicular plate of the nasal septum), the middle turbinate remnant, and the olfactory cleft bilaterally. The dura is elevated laterally off the orbital roof to facilitate placement of the composite tissue graft during endoscopic reconstruction of the skull-base defect. Also, the anterior and posterior ethmoidal arteries are cauterized with a bipolar or monopolar cautery. A wide dural margin is resected extending anteroposteriorly from the posterior wall of the frontal sinus to the optic chiasm. Laterally, the dural margin is initially resected a few millimeters medial to the junction of the orbital wall and the ethmoid roof. The dura, bilateral cribriform plate with olfactory bulbs, middle turbinate remnant, perpendicular plate of the septum, and the inferior crista galli are removed *en bloc* through the nose as a final specimen. Smaller lesions limited to the olfactory cleft are resected in a similar fashion, but with sparing of the contralateral septal mucosa, cribriform plate, and paranasal sinuses.

After the resection is complete, adjacent brain parenchyma and the intracranial cavity are inspected for the presence of neoplasm, and frozen sections are sent circumferentially from the dural margins, olfactory nerve endings, and septum. Additional margins are sent as needed. Endoscopic marsupialization of the lacrimal sac is performed with a cutting forceps or powered instrumentation to minimize the chance of subsequent stenosis and secondary epiphora. Bipolar cautery is used to control any bleeding meningeal vessels. Endoscopic repair of the final anterior skull-base defect generally requires a composite reconstruction utilizing a wide variety of autoplastic and/or alloplastic materials (103–105).

References

1. Miculitz JV. Zut operativen behandlung des empyems der highmorshohle. Zeitschr für Heilk. 7,4. Ileft, 1886.
2. Halle M. Die intranasalen operationen bei eitrigen erkrankungen der nebenhohlen der nase. *Arch Laryngol Rhinol* 1915; 29:73–112.
3. Mosher HP. The surgical anatomy of the ethmoidal labyrinth. *Ann Otol Rhinol Laryngol* 1929; 38:869–901.
4. Van Alyea OE. The ostium maxillare: anatomic study of its surgical accessibility. *Arch Otolaryngol* 1936; 24:553–569.
5. Van Alyea OE. Ethmoid labyrinth: anatomic study, with consideration of the clinical significance of its structural characteristics. *Arch Otolaryngol* 1939; 29(6):881–902.
6. Van Alyea OE. Sphenoid sinus: anatomic study, with consideration of the clinical significance of the structural characteristics of the sphenoid sinus. *Arch Otolaryngol* 1941; 34:225–253.
7. Van Alyea OE. Nasal Sinuses: An Anatomic and Clinical Consideration. Baltimore: Williams & Wilkins, 1951.
8. Myerson M. The natural orifice of the maxillary sinus. I. Anatomic studies. *Arch Otolaryngol* 1932; 15:80–91.
9. Hajek M. Pathologie und therapie der entzundlichen erkrankungen der nebenhohlen der nase. 5th ed. Leipzig: Deuticke, 1926.
10. Neivert H. Surgical anatomy of the maxillary sinus. *Laryngoscope* 1930; 40:1–4.
11. Draf W. Endoscopy of the Paranasal Sinuses. New York: Springer-Verlag, 1983.

12. Maltz M. New instrument: the sinuscope. *Laryngoscope* 1925; 35:805–811.

13. Messerklinger W. Uber die drainage der menschlichen nasennebenholen unter normalen und pathologischen bendingungen II: die stirnhole und ihr ausfuhrungssystem. *Monatsschr Ohrenheilkd* 1967; 101:313–326.

14. Messerklinger W. Endosckopiche diagnose und chirurgie der rezidivierenden sinusitis. In: *Krajina Z, ed. Advances in Nose and Sinus Surgery*. Zagreb, Yugoslavia: Zagreb University; 1985.

15. Naumann H. Pathologische anatomie der chronischen rhinitis und sinusitis. In: *Proceedings VIII International Congress of Oto-Rhinolaryngology*. Amsterdam, the Netherlands: Excerpta Medica, 1965:80.

16. Stamberger H. Endoscopic endonasal surgery—concepts in treatment of recurring rhinosinusitis. Part I. Anatomic and pathophysiologic considerations. *Otolaryngol Head Neck Surg* 1986; 94:143–147.

17. Stamberger H. Endoscopic endonasal surgery: concepts in treatment of recurring rhinosinusitis. Part II. Surgical technique. *Otolaryngol Head Neck Surg* 1986; 94:147–56.

18. Wigand ME, Steiner W, Jaumann MP. Endonasal sinus surgery with endoscopical control from radical operation to rehabilitation of the mucosa. *Endoscopy (Stuttg)* 1978; 10:255–60.

19. Wigand ME. Transnasal ethmoidectomy under endoscopical control. *Rhinology* 1981; 19:7–15.

20. Wigand ME. Endoscopic surgery of the paranasal sinuses and anterior skull base. New York, NY: Thieme Medical Publishers, 1990.

21. Draf W. Die chirurgische behandlung entzundlicher erkrankungen der nasennebenhohlen. *Arch Otorhinoalaryngol* 1982; 235:133–305.

22. Kennedy DW, Zinreich SJ, Rosenbaum AE, et al. Functional endoscopic sinus surgery. Theory and diagnostic evaluation. *Arch Otolaryngol* 1985; 111:576–82.

23. Rice DH, Schaefer SD. Endoscopic paranasal sinus surgery. New York NY: Raven Press, 1988.

24. Rice DH. Basic surgical techniques and variations of endoscopic sinus surgery. *Otolaryngol Clin North Am* 1989; 22:713–26.

25. Schaefer SD. Endoscopic total sphenoethmoidectomy. *Otolaryngol Clin North Am* 1989; 22:727–32.

26. Schaefer SD. An anatomic approach to endoscopic intranasal ethmoidectomy. *Laryngoscope* 1998; 108;1628–34.

27. May M, Schaitkin B, Kay SL. Revision endoscopic sinus surgery: six friendly surgical landmarks. *Laryngoscope* 1994; 104(6):766–767.

28. May M, Sobol SM, Korzec K. The location of the maxillary os and its importance to the endoscopic sinus surgeon. *Laryngoscope* 1990; 100(10):1037–1042.

29. Parsons D, Bolger W, Boyd E. The "ridge"—a safer entry to the sphenoid sinus during functional endoscopic sinus surgery in children. *Operative Tech Otolaryngol Head Neck Surg* 1994; 5:43–4.

30. Bolger W, Keyes AS, Lanza DC. Use of the superior meatus and superior turbinate in the endoscopic approach to the sphenoid sinus. *Otolaryngol Head Neck Surg* 1999; 20(3):308–13.

31. Hosemann W, Gross R, Gode U, et al. The anterior sphenoid wall: relative anatomy for sphenoidotomy. *Am J Rhinol* 1995; 9:137–44.

32. Stankiewicz JA. The endoscopic approach to the sphenoid sinus. *Laryngoscope* 1989; 99:218–221.

33. Casiano RR. Correlation of clinical examination with computer tomography in paranasal sinus disease. *Am J Rhinol* 1997;11(3):193–6.

34. Ritter FN. The Paranasal Sinuses: Anatomy and Surgical Technique. 2nd ed. St. Louis: CV Mosby, 1978.

35. Lang J. Clinical Anatomy of the Nose, Nasal Cavity and the Paranasal Sinuses. New York: Thieme Medical Publishers, 1989.

36. Calhoun KH, Rotzler WH, Stiernberg CM. Surgical anatomy of the lateral nasal wall. *Otolaryngol Head Neck Surg* 1990; 102:156–160.

37. Casiano RR. A stepwise surgical technique using the medial orbital floor as the key landmark in performing endoscopic sinus surgery. *Laryngoscope* 2001; 111(6):964–974.

38. Friedman M, Tanyeri H, Lim J, Landsberg R, Caldarelli D. A safe, alternative technique for inferior turbinate reduction. *Laryngoscope* 1999; 109(11):1834–1837.

39. Van delden MR, Cook PR, Davis WE. Endoscopic partial inferior turbinoplasty. *Otolaryngol Head Neck Surg* 1999; 121(4):406–409.

40. Passali D, Lauriello M, Anselmi M, Bellussi L. Treatment of hypertrophy of the inferior turbinate: long-term results in 382 patients randomly assigned to therapy. *Ann Otol Rhinol Laryngol* 1999;108(6):569–575.

41. Berenholz L, Kessler A, Sarfati S, Eviatar E, Segal S. Chronic sinusitis: a sequela of inferior turbinectomy. *Am J Rhinol* 1998; 12(4):257–261.

42. Hwang PH, McLaughlin RB, Lanza DC, Kennedy DW. Endoscopic septoplasty: indications, technique, and results. *Otolaryngol Head Neck Surg* 1999; 120(5):678–682.

43. Nayak DR, Balakrishnan R, Murthy KD. An endoscopic approach to the deviated nasal septum—a preliminary study. *J Laryngol Otol* 1998; 112(10):934–939.

44. Yanagisawa E, Joe J. Endoscopic septoplasty. *Ear Nose Throat J* 1997; 76(9):622–623.

45. Giles WC, Gross CW, Abram AC, Greene WM, Avner TG. Endoscopic septoplasty. *Laryngoscope* 1994; 104(12):1507–1509.

46. Havas TE, Lowinger DS. Comparison of functional endonasal sinus surgery with and without partial middle turbinate resection. *Ann Otol Rhinol Laryngol* 2000; 109(7):634–640.

47. Banfield GK, McCombe A. Partial resection of the middle turbinate at functional endoscopic sinus surgery. *J R Army Med Corps* 1999; 145(1):18–19.

48. Giacchi RJ, Lebowitz RA, Jacobs JB. Middle turbinate resection: issues and controversies. *Am J Rhinol* 2000; 14(3):193–197.

49. Fortune DS, Duncavage JA. Incidence of frontal sinusitis following partial middle turbinectomy. *Ann Otol Rhinol Laryngol* 1998; 107(6):447–453.

50. Lee WC, Ming Ku PK, van Hasselt CA. New guidelines for endoscopic localization of the anterior ethmoidal artery: a cadaveric study. *Laryngoscope* 2000; 110(7):1173–1178.

51. Budrovich R, Saetti R.Microscopic and endoscopic ligature of the sphenopalatine artery. *Laryngoscope* 1992; 102(12 Pt 1):1391–1394.

52. Sharp HR, Rowe-Jones JM, Biring GS, Mackay IS. Endoscopic ligation or diathermy of the sphenopalatine artery in persistent epistaxis. *J Laryngol Otol* 1997; 111(11):1047–1050.

53. Srinivasan V, Sherman IW, O'Sullivan G. Surgical management of intractable epistaxis: audit of results. *J Laryngol Otol* 2000; 114(9):697–700.

54. Carrau RL, Snyderman CH, Kassam AB, Jungreis CA. Endoscopic and endoscopic-assisted surgery for juvenile angiofibroma. *Laryngoscope* 2001; 111(3):483–487.

55. Tseng HZ, Chao WY. Transnasal endoscopic approach for juvenile nasopharyngeal angiofibroma. *Am J Otolaryngol* 1997; 18:151–154.

56. Fagan JJ, Snyderman CH, Carrau RL, et al. Nasopharyngeal angiofibromas: selecting a surgical approach. *Head Neck* 1997; 19:391–399.

57. Ungkanont K, Byers RM, Weber RS, et al. Juvenile nasopharyngeal angiofibroma: an update of therapeutic management. *Head Neck* 1996; 18:60–66.

58. Wareing MJ, Padgham ND. Osteologic classification of the sphenopalatine foramen. *Laryngoscope* 1998; 108(1 Pt 1):125–127.

59. Woolford TJ, Jones NS. Endoscopic ligation of anterior ethmoidal artery in treatment of epistaxis. *J Laryngol Otol* 2000; 114(11):858–860.

60. Metternich FU, Brusis T. [Ethmoid sinus operation for therapy of recurrence severe epistaxis.] *Laryngorhinootologie* 1998; 77(10):582–586.

61. Cokkeser Y, Evereklioglu C, Er H. Comparative external versus endoscopic dacryocystorhinostomy results in 115 patients (130 eyes). *Otolaryngol Head Neck Surg* 2000; 123(4):488–491.

62. Szubin L, Papageorge A, Sacks E. Endonasal laser-assisted dacryocystorhinostomy. *Am J Rhinol* 1999; 13(5):371–374.

63. Hartikainen J, Antila J, Varpula M, Puukka P, Seppa H, Grenman R. Prospective randomized comparison of endonasal endoscopic dacryocystorhinostomy and external dacryocystorhinostomy. *Laryngoscope* 1998; 108(12):1861–1866.

64. Hehar SS, Jones NS, Sadiq SA, Downes RN. Endoscopic holmium:YAG laser dacryocystorhinostomy-safe and effective as a day-case procedure. *J Laryngol Otol* 1997; 111(11):1056–1059.

65. Sprekelsen MB, Barberan MT. Endoscopic dacryocystorhinostomy: surgical technique and results. *Laryngoscope* 1996; 106(2 Pt 1):187–189.

66. Metson R, Woog JJ, Puliafito CA. Endoscopic laser dacryocystorhinostomy. *Laryngoscope* 1994; 104(3 Pt 1):269–274.

67. Wormald PJ, Kew J, Van Hasselt A. Intranasal anatomy of the nasolacrimal sac in endoscopic dacryocystorhinostomy. *Otolaryngol Head Neck Surg* 2000; 123(3):307–310.

68. Yung MW, Logan BM. The anatomy of the lacrimal bone at the lateral wall of the nose: its significance to the lacrimal surgeon. *Clin Otolaryngol* 1999; 24(4):262–265.

69. Kessler A, Berenholz LP, Segal S. Transnasal endoscopic drainage of a medial subperiosteal orbital abscess. *Eur Arch Otorhinolaryngol* 1998; 255(6):293–295.

70. Page EL, Wiatrak BJ. Endoscopic vs external drainage of orbital subperiosteal abscess. *Arch Otolaryngol Head Neck Surg* 1996; 122(7):737–740.

71. Deutsch E, Eilon A, Hevron I, Hurvitz H, Blinder G. Functional endoscopic sinus surgery of orbital subperiosteal abscess in children. *Int J Pediatr Otorhinolaryngol* 1996; 34(1-2):181–190.

72. Manning SC. Endoscopic management of medial subperiosteal orbital abscess. *Arch Otolaryngol Head Neck Surg* 1993; 119(7):789–791.

73. Ulualp SO, Massaro BM, Toohill RJ. Course of proptosis in patients with Graves' disease after endoscopic orbital decompression. *Laryngoscope* 1999; 109(8):1217–1222.

74. Graham SM, Carter KD. Combined-approach orbital decompression for thyroid-related orbitopathy. *Clin Otolaryngol* 1999; 24(2):109–113.

75. Shepard KG, Levin PS, Terris DJ. Balanced orbital decompression for Graves' ophthalmopathy. *Laryngoscope* 1998; 108(11 Pt 1):1648–1653.

76. Lund VJ, Larkin G, Fells P, Adams G. Orbital decompression for thyroid eye disease: a comparison of external and endoscopic techniques. J Laryngol Otol 1997; 111(1):1051–1055.

77. Koay B, Bates G, Elston J. Endoscopic orbital decompression for dysthyroid eye disease. *J Laryngol Otol* 1997; 111(10):946–949.

78. Metson R, Shore JW, Gliklich RE, Dallow RL. Endoscopic orbital decompression under local anesthesia. *Otolaryngol Head Neck Surg* 1995; 113(6):661–667.

79. Kennedy DW, Goodstein ML, Miller NR, Zinreich SJ. Endoscopic transnasal orbital decompression. *Arch Otolaryngol Head Neck Surg* 1990; 116(3):275–282.

80. Wright ED, Davidson J, Codere F, Desrosiers M. Endoscopic orbital decompression with preservation of an inferomedial bony strut: minimization fo postoperative diplopia. *J Otolaryngol* 1999; 28(5):252–256.

81. Lee WC. Recurrent frontal sinusitis complicating orbital decompression in Graves' disease. *J Laryngol Otol* 1996; 110(7):670–672.

82. Bough ID, Huang JJ, Pribitkin EA. Orbital decompression for Graves' disease complicated by sinusitis. *Ann Otol Rhinol Laryngol* 1994; 103(12):988–990.

83. Kountakis SE, Maillard AA, El-Harazi SM, Longhini L, Urso RG. Endoscopic optic nerve decompression for traumatic blindness. *Otolaryngol Head Neck Surg* 2000; 123(1 Pt 1):34–37.

84. Luxenberger W, Stammberger H, Jebeles JA, Walch C. Endoscopic optic nerve decompression: the Graz experience. *Laryngoscope* 1998; 108(6):873–882.

85. Graham SM, Carter KD. Combined endoscopic and subciliary orbital decompression for thyroid-related compressive optic neuropathy. *Rhinology* 1997; 35(3):103–107.

86. Kuppersmith RB, Alford EL, Patrinely JR, Lee AG, Parke RB, Holds JB. Combined transconjunctival/intranasal endoscopic approach to the optic canal in traumatic optic neuropathy. *Laryngoscope* 1997; 107(3):311–315.

87. Ulualp SO, Carlson TK, Toohill RJ. Osteoplastic flap versus modified endoscopic Lothrop procedure in patients with frontal sinus disease. *Am J Rhinol* 2000; 14(1):21–26.

88. Kikawada T, Fujigaki M, Kikura M, Matsumoto M, Kikawada k. Extended endoscopic frontal sinus surgery to interrupted nasofrontal communication caused by scarring of the anterior ethmoid: long-term results. *Arch Otolaryngol Head Neck Surg* 1999; 125(1):92–96.

89. Casiano RR, Livingston JA. Endoscopic Lothrop procedure. *Am J Rhinol* 1998; 12(5):335–339.

90. Gross CW, Zachman GC, Becker DG, Vickery CL, Moore DF Jr, Lindsey WH, Gross WE. Follow-up of University of Virginia experience with the modified Lothrop procedure. *Am J Rhinol* 1997; 11(1):49–54.

91. McLaughlin RB, Hwang PH, Lanza DC. Endoscopic trans-septal frontal sinusotomy: the rationale and results of an alternative technique. *Am J Rhinol* 1999; 13(4):279–287.

92. Lund VJ. Optimum management of inverted papilloma. *J Laryngol Otol* 2000; 114(3):194–197.

93. Sukenic MA, Casiano R. Endoscopic medial maxillectomy for inverted papillomas of the paranasal sinuses: value of the intraoperative endoscopic examination. *Laryngoscope* 2000; 110(1):39–42.

94. Chee LW, Sethi DS. The endoscopic management of sinonasal inverted papillomas. *Clin Otolaryngol* 1999; 24(1):61–66.

95. Tufano RP; Thaler ER, Lanza DC, Goldberg AN, Kennedy DW: Endoscopic management of sinonasal inverted papilloma. *Am J Rhinol* 1999; 13(6):423–426.

96. Kamel RH. Transnasal endoscopic medial maxillectomy in inverted papilloma. *Laryngoscope* 1995; 105(8 Pt 1):847–853.

97. Stankiewicz JA, Girgis SJ. Endoscopic surgical treatment of nasal and paranasal sinus inverted papilloma. *Otolaryngol Head Neck Surg* 1993; 109(6):988–995.

98. Koren I, Hadar T, Rappaport ZH, Yaniv E. Endoscopic transnasal transsphenoidal microsurgery versus the sublabial approach for the treatment of pituitary tumors:endonasal complications. *Laryngoscope* 1999; 109(11):1838–1840.

99. Nasseri SS, McCaffrey TV, Kasperbauer JL, Atkinson JL. A combined, minimally invasive transnasal approach to the sella turcica. *Am J Rhinol* 1998; 12(6):409–16.

100. Aust MR, McCaffrey TV, Atkinson J. Transnasal endoscopic approach to the sella turcica. *Am J Rhinol* 1998; 12(4):283–287.